A BREACH
OF TRUST

Susan Hodges, LNFA

ISBN: 1517481244
ISBN 13: 9781517481247

DEDICATION

To my sons, who gave me the greatest gift of my life—my grandkids.

To my big sister, Linda Ann, who held my hand all the way through our mother Katie's passing, and to this date still hasn't let go.

I will always remember the dedicated service of each DON, ADON, LVN, CNA, BOM, MDS director, medical director, social service worker, activity director, therapist, maintenance director & assistants, dietary director & aides, housekeeper/floor tech, laundry director & aides, and all the consultants in the nursing home. I had such joy working with all of you. You are truly my heroes. *Hugs.*

This is also for the late Tommy and Kate Gay. Dad, thanks for feeding me food from the garden you planted. Mom, thanks for setting your table with the most wonderful garden dishes—fresh black eyed peas, tomatoes, fried okra, squash, fresh onions and peppers, and of course, corn on the cob. I am forever grateful for our family meals, where love and encouragement was always abundant.

To all above: "I would tell you I love you from the bottom of my heart, but with you my heart has no bottom." *~ author unknown*

Susan Hodges

To the reader:

You are about to read a true story, though many obstacles had to be cleared before these words could be put down into print. First, HIPAA prevents the release of all information regarding patients and/or residents when it involves healthcare. As a result, I had to change the names and backgrounds of all of the patients/residents. To be safe, I then had to create a fictitious location for the nursing home, as well as fictitious names for the several other nursing homes involved in this story. The next hurdle required me to change the names of all of the people involved except for me. Even though some of them are public figures and the story is true, I didn't want to risk identifying any of the characters. Finally, to keep the lawyers happy, I had to change the order of some events to continue this 'real person protection,' as well as to help the story flow better. I have read about writers producing creative fiction and while there are some creative aspects to this book, I consider it fully a true story, one produced from my memory and personal experiences. It is not a style of work called 'creative nonfiction.' With all of that said, I hope you both enjoy the story and are better informed when you have completed this book. You can contact me at ABreachofTrust2016@gmail.com with any questions or comments.

Thanks!

Susan Hodges, LNFA

PROLOGUE

I t was a bright, cool day—a spring day—a day to be outside tasting the crispness of the air, delighting in the scent of the season's first blossoms. Every year Fort Worth experienced many of these days and each time it did, the people were happier. They'd graciously let you move your car ahead of them and didn't honk when you failed to signal. They'd smile in the grocery store parking lot and sometimes even help you with your bags. Spring brought forth hope, for we knew that soon the landscape would be adorned in brilliant colors and gentle scents. The air whispered tidings of the life that would soon be bursting from both earth and tree. For most folks in the North Texas area, it was a great time to be alive.

As for me, perhaps two or three times a year I left my workplace at the stroke of noon, climbed into my Chevy, and drove to lunch somewhere. What was even rarer than eating out for lunch, was the special occasion of getting a hot dog. Today I was going to do it all. And I had the perfect place picked out, a place I'd been to a few times already.

I worked at the Jones-Simms Nursing Center. It was a licensed skilled nursing home located in a very rough part of Fort Worth. I was its Licensed Nursing Facility Administrator (LNFA). That basically meant I was the CEO. Directly or indirectly everyone answered to me, and I was responsible for everyone and everything. Believe me, the state of Texas made sure of that!

As I pulled out of the parking lot, a brief scan of the building and parking lot showed nothing out of place. It was a good omen. I drove away in a great mood with my windows rolled down, sniffing the scents in the air, and enjoying that perfect mixture of cool-yet-not-cold breeze on my face.

Even though the area was rough, somehow today it didn't seem so bad. Perhaps even the gang members were taking a holiday. How could anyone do anything wrong on a day like this? I know, wishful thinking. But on a day like today it was hard to think of anything dark or dirty or criminal.

The restaurant I was going to was almost twenty minutes away. It was longer than I felt comfortable with, but a while back a friend of mine had told me about their steaming soft buns, piping hot turkey dogs, stiff yellow mustard, and the meaty chili piled along one side. Quite frankly, I had to have one. And my first few trips there hadn't disappointed.

The drive took me through the rougher parts of Fort Worth and into the nicer areas, where I reached Big Dogs and found a parking spot near the back of the restaurant. The place was positively packed. When I opened the glass door, the smell of fresh buns, onions and chili hit my nose. The line nearly reached the door, but I was expecting it. I took my place at the end of the line and filed in behind a young couple. Several more people joined the line behind me, all wearing relaxed, pleasant smiles on their faces. Again, no one was allowed to be upset today, including me.

I'd been in line for about two minutes when I heard the traditional ring of a phone from a bygone era. It was my cell phone. The loud ringer turned a few heads, but no one seemed upset. I quickly removed it from my purse and looked at the number. It was from work.

I'm gone barely twenty minutes and they feel the need to call me. Well, it's time for some tough love.

I pushed the switch down and put the phone on vibrate. Whatever it was could wait until I got back. I had good people working for me—at some point they needed to learn to solve problems on their own. Besides, this was a rare treat and I wasn't going to let them ruin it for me.

It took almost ten minutes to get to the counter, where I ordered my hot dog and a soft drink and slid down the counter, waiting for someone to make it. The smells from the kitchen had my mouth watering, even though I'd already been salivating all the way on the drive over. Once I'd paid and collected my tray, I found an open seat at a bar that faced a window with an unobstructed view of the high-way and its traffic. Even that didn't bother me.

Just when I was about to tear in to my hot dog, a loud rattling sounded from within the depths of my purse. The phone was up against my car keys and the whole affair lay on the hard counter, giving the vibrate setting a ringtone of its own. I shook the purse and it stopped. Still, a minute later I could hear the phone vibrating again. Whoever it was, they couldn't take a hint. Well tough. I was having some *me* time.

I ate my meal, savoring each bite. When I was done, I sipped idly on my soda and did some car watching. Many of the vehicles looked like they were coming from the fancy car wash down the street. A few still dripped water from their wheel wells. Occasionally a pedestrian walked by, giving me a chance to study them. I amused myself for a while trying to guess what they did for a living and where they might have come from. When my soda ran dry, I grabbed my purse and exited the store, taking in a deep breath and enjoying the clean, fresh Texas air.

Reaching into the purse, I felt for my car keys. Just as I did, my phone vibrated.

Oh for crying out loud, who could be calling so many times?!

I pulled the phone out and looked at the display: WORK 5 Missed Calls. I opened the car door and sat down on the driver's seat, resignedly pressing the voicemail button.

Beep. Message One. "Susan, this is Cayla. Some male CNAs (Certified Nursing Assistants) just showed up in three different vans. They say they're from other nursing homes and they're here to take away Gracie, Dale and Ari. I asked them to wait for you, but they said they're not waiting for anybody. Please call me back."

Beep. Message Two. "Susan, please call me right now! They've grabbed Gracie and she's putting up a fight. Some of the residents are helping her resist. They're lifting her out of her chair forcibly. It's terrible. Call me!"

Beep. Message Three. "Susan, two CNAs are grabbing Ari. A nurse is trying to stop them, I'm trying to . . . *hey*! PUT HIM DOWN NOW! Hey mister you're going to be . . ."

Beep. Message Four. "Susan for the love of God, HURRY BACK! The residents are crying and screaming. (I could hear chaos in the background.) This is horrible to watch. It's something straight out of a nightmare. (She was crying now.) I can't stop them. They're too strong. They're storm troopers. No warning, no paperwork, they're just kidnapping these sweet people."

Beep. Message Five. "Susan, it's bad. (Deep sobbing.) PLEASE CALL ME. PLEASE HURRY!" *Beep*. End of messages.

Suddenly the spring air was stale and the pleasant meal I'd just eaten threatened to be eaten once more. My heart felt like it was exploding, beating rapidly as I dropped the phone, jammed the key into the ignition and fired up my Chevy. Then, for probably the first time in life, I peeled out of the parking lot with tires smoking. I prayed to God I wouldn't be too late.

1

Five years earlier

"Susan, I need to talk to you in my office when you have a moment."

"Certainly Ms. Hightower, just let me gather up my things and I'll be right in." As Ms. Hightower walked away, I hoped it would be good news. I was only days away from completing the course requirements needed to obtain my state license, and I was hoping to be a bona fide administrator for some well-respected nursing home in Texas sooner rather than later. The only thing that stood in my way was a six-month internship under the supervision of a qualified Preceptor (LNFA with at least five years of skilled nursing experience). Tarrant County Community College arranged the placements for us and Ms. Hightower was the Internship Placement Director. Brimming with excitement, I quickly gathered up my things and made my way to her office.

Tapping on her slightly ajar door, I said, "Ms. Hightower, are you ready to see me?"

"Yes. Please have a seat."

Ms. Hightower sat behind her desk, holding an open folder. Taking a seat, I set my things on the floor and folded my hands, nervously waiting for her to speak.

"Susan, we've been able to find a spot for you here in Fort Worth, so you won't have to be driving too far. We've also managed to land you a spot with *the* premier nursing facility in Fort Worth, and I daresay, all of Texas. Of course, your excellent grades and maturity certainly played a big role in their acceptance of you."

My heart raced. *A premier nursing facility.* This would be the perfect place to learn all the best procedures and latest in technology. What a dream come true!

"Thank you so much! Where will I be working?"

"It's called the Wellington Hills Home and it's located downtown. I think you'll find the buildings and grounds extraordinary. Really, this is the best of the best. And I don't say that lightly. Neither the poor, nor the middle class people in Fort Worth will be in this facility. Not even most of the wealthy. Only the people *they* think are wealthy are the ones who can afford this facility. We're rarely able to place an intern there, but you being fifty-six years old helped out a lot. You'll still have to do an interview with the LNFA there and be approved before it's official, though. I have an appointment set up for tomorrow. Here's the time and the address. Susan, I know you'll dress appropriately and represent TCC well. Please call and let me know if you're approved so I can add it to your file. Any questions?"

"No, Ms. Hightower. I'm ever so grateful for your confidence in me and I'll do everything in my power to please the LNFA, I assure you."

She closed the file, rose to her feet and shook my hand. "I'm sure you will, Susan. Good luck."

I was totally on cloud nine. I hadn't heard of Wellington Hills Home before, but that was no surprise. Most of my class couldn't even name one nursing facility beyond the two we'd visited during our coursework. The fact that it was for the super-wealthy made it even more unlikely any of us had ever heard of it. As soon as I got home I did some research on the place so as to be as prepared as possible. Afterwards I selected a nice outfit, ironed it and waited eagerly for the next day to come.

I arrived the next morning a full thirty minutes early. This gave me the opportunity to check out the grounds and gather my first impression. Unfortunately, there wasn't much to see. The ten-story building itself was nondescript, and along with various other structures, blocked the view of the grounds. I assumed this was because they didn't want the residents sitting by the pool staring at passing traffic or wandering off. With nothing but roofs, large trees and buildings to see, I found a bench and waited for the time to tick off.

With two minutes to spare, I walked into the ornate lobby and approached the front desk.

"May I help you?" the receptionist asked.

"Yes, I'm Susan Hodges and I have an appointment with Ms. Greenwald."

"Of course. Let me ring her."

I looked around the lobby as she dialed the extension. During my lifetime, I'd only seen two ways of displaying wealth: tastefully or gaudily. At this very moment I was experiencing a third kind: opulently. Each carving, statue, painting and piece of furniture cost more than my entire lifetime earnings, yet it was displayed and arranged in such a way that went beyond tasteful. Opulent is the only word I can use to describe it. The floor was made of some rare marble and beautifully integrated with a combination of complex wall coverings and painted finishes. I won't even say 'faux' finishes since there was nothing *faux* about it. If I were a super rich person thinking about placing Mom here or even staying here myself, I'd certainly feel beyond comfortable with this first impression.

The receptionist hung up the phone. "Ms. Greenwald's assistant will be here in a moment to show you in."

"Thank you," I replied.

A few seconds later the solid wood door opened up and a young woman approached. "Ms. Hodges, I'm Deborah. I'll take you to see Ms. Greenwald."

"Thank you," I said, following her through the door.

She moved next to me and said, "Ms. Greenwald's office is actually right next to the reception area, but I wanted to take you along the path we show all visitors and potential residents to get you acquainted with the facility."

"Thank you, that would be nice."

"The building is ten stories tall with the residents occupying the upper nine floors. When they're healthy and mobile, they start out on the upper five floors. As they need more help, we move them down to assisted living on floors three through five. Once they're confined to bed or on hospice, they're moved down to the second floor."

"I see. Very efficient."

"The ground floor is where we have all of the common areas. The building is actually a perfect square—we have four long halls along the perimeter, each with a different theme. This one is our Italian-themed hall called Tuscany. Here we have wine cellars for the residents to store their collections, as well as the facility's. We also have various rooms for board meetings. Each room has full A/V technology and is capable of video conferencing. It's also where we hold lectures for guest speakers or project them from overseas via video."

I studied the walls and floors and knew without a doubt that everything had been imported directly from Italy. No detail had been overlooked. It was very impressive.

"Now we're in Burgundy, the French hall. Here we have more meeting rooms, places for art instruction, and of course, entertainment."

Like the Italian hall before, this French-themed hall had everything imported directly from France. Several tables even held fresh, massive sunflowers!

When we turned another corner, she said, "This is the American hall. We call it Independence. As you can see, it's mostly a colonial decor with an actual handwritten copy of the Declaration of Independence made in 1776 there on the wall. This is where we house our movie theatre, along with two different eating rooms which we sometimes use instead of the big one in the next hall."

Mounted on the walls were real muskets, which I was sure appealed to the same independent thinkers who made the money to afford to stay in such a place. Just walking through this hall and seeing the paintings of the War of Independence made me want to join up with General Washington's army right then and there!

"This last hall is my favorite. Of course, it's the Texas hall and we've named it the Chisholm Trail for the cattle trail that actually goes right through Fort Worth. Here we have our staff offices, a large dining area, and a few more meeting rooms."

The walls were decorated with cowboy and cattle paraphernalia, with a few oil derricks tossed in. It was both comfortable and inviting.

"Here we are at Ms. Greenwald's office." We walked into a relatively small secretarial area (which was Deborah's) and then into Mrs. Greenwald's larger office, which was also decorated in a Texas theme. She had a small table to the side where she sat reviewing my file.

"Ms. Hodges," she said shaking my hand. "It's a pleasure to meet you. Please, have a seat. Deborah, please hold my calls."

"Certainly, Ms. Greenwald. Ms. Hodges, may I get you something to drink? We have several kinds of bottled water: Fiji, Evian, Pellegrino and, of course, Perrier. We also have an assortment of soft drinks and freshly squeezed juices."

"No, thank you. I'm perfectly fine."

"Certainly," she replied, and she left us to our meeting.

"So Susan, I have several questions for you but first, why did you get into nursing home care this late in life? Your resume says you're fifty-six."

I cleared my throat, prepared for questions like this one. "Several years ago, my father developed cancer. I wanted to know what to expect and what the effects of his type of cancer would do to his body and mind. I felt that understanding this would help me take better care of him and make sure he received the best treatment possible. While I was researching his type of cancer, I had a friend who was an administrator of a hospital tell me, 'If you want to learn about it, you should go back to college and take some medical courses.' So I did, and I ended up liking the several nursing home courses I took, even though I started out trying to learn more about my father's disease and how I could help him along medically. Then I took a few more nursing home courses and before long, I wanted to be an LNFA. So really, it all just sort of happened because of my father."

"I see. That's a very unique answer, one I don't believe I've ever heard before. For someone to do something like that for their parents . . . it's very loving. How's your father doing?"

"He recently passed away."

Ms. Greenwald's demeanor changed. "Oh, I'm sorry. After losing him, do you still want to make this a career?"

"Definitely. I truly love the business, or at least what I've seen so far."

"That's good," she said, lowering her eyes to my resume. "I've been looking over your background and it's also very interesting. You were a property manager for twenty years, both residential and commercial. Tell me more about that."

"Yes, I had great clients like 7-Eleven, Stop'n Go, Mercedes Benz, and Baskin Robbins. They all needed offices and hired my company to handle their remodels and rehabs. I also managed a six-story building and four strip centers. After that, I managed a residential complex. It was a good career."

"Yes, it sure sounds like it. And I see you have two sons?"

"Three actually, because I count my step-son from my second marriage. I married young and got divorced after just two years. Then I met the love of my life. He had a heart attack on our driveway and I wasn't there to help him. My six-year-old son was there and called my mother, who drove over, picked him up and raced him to the ER. Still, he died five days later. I still think about him often, even though it all happened over twenty years ago."

"I understand," she said pushing back from the table a bit. "You have great grades and the maturity we're interested in. You understand this is a six-month AIT position (Administrator in Training) and you will not be paid."

"Yes, I know that. It's part of the state's licensing requirements."

"That's right. All we can offer you is hard work, excellent experience and possibly a good reference, *if* you do well."

"I'm ready for it, Ms. Greenwald. Just give me a chance."

She studied the resume for a few more seconds, and then smiled at me. "Well Susan, I think we're going to take you on. And I don't say that lightly. We rarely take on interns because of the high status of our facility. We can't afford to have folks that don't know what they're doing—our clients are quite exclusive and expect only the best. They trust us. Our waiting list is extensive and once someone finally makes it in, they have to pay a minimum $250,000 for a 600 sq. ft. room or smaller. This fee is nonrefundable and not inheritable. Of course, many pay more for larger, more comfortable accommodations."

"Wow! I didn't know that. I promise, I won't let you down!"

"Yes, I'm sure you won't. I'm going to start you on the second floor, which is Skilled Nursing. That's where you'll get the most experience for wherever you land as an LNFA." She stood up and shook my hand again. "I'm going to send you off with Deborah. She'll get you organized. Any questions?"

"No, I'm just very excited for this opportunity. I greatly appreciate it."

Deborah came in and escorted me out of the office. A few minutes later I was belted in my car travelling home and carrying a head filled with amazement.

"I got the internship and I start tomorrow!"

"Wonderful and congratulations!" the voice said. "Aren't you the lucky one! I've got an interview at a place in Granbury, and assuming I get it, that's a long haul for me each day. It's a rural-type place—a far cry from the fancy digs you landed."

I was talking to Vicki, a friend I'd met in our classes at TCC. She, along with seven other LNFA students, also needed to complete a six-month AIT internship. After that, we could all start getting paid to run a nursing home, assuming we could find one to hire us.

"I may be lucky now," I told her, "but in six months all of our slates are wiped clean. We'll all be competing for any open LNFA positions in the North Texas area."

"That's true. Then it's game on. But at least you'll have Wellington Hills on your resume. I'll just have some podunk home in Granbury. I like your chances better than mine."

"Oh, stop complaining. You're just trying to sandbag me into feeling sorry for you and then you'll be the first one to get a job."

"Maybe," she said laughing. "But at least we can both celebrate your good fortune, right?

I giggled. "Sure, but let me get a week in first and then we'll meet up. Deal?"

"Deal! And if I get this internship, we can compare notes."

"Good idea. Talk to you then."

I hung up the phone and began making preparations for my first day of work at Wellington Hills. I wanted everything to be perfect.

When I arrived, the first thing Deborah did was take me on a complete tour of the grounds. First, she showed me the exterior which included the swimming pool area. It looked like something out of Las Vegas: cascading waterfalls, hot tubs, wading pools—the works! Several women were already in the pool taking a water aerobics class. Deborah knew each resident and addressed them by their surnames, "Hello, Mrs. Johnson. How are you doing today, Mrs. Jones?" They each knew her name, too. Everything was very family-like.

Next to the pool was a putting green. It wasn't large, but it was certainly more than adequate. Both the putting green and pool area were open to the sky, yet sheltered by trees, bushes, and maintenance buildings from the adjoining office buildings. It was certainly a nice set up.

After looking over all of this, Deborah took me to an aviary filled with hundreds of birds. An employee was putting special grain in several containers and making sure the self-feeding water supply was working. Deborah explained that the man was an ornithologist and held a class each week for the residents to learn about different species of birds. By now, I wasn't surprised.

After we completed a tour of the grounds, we went inside and explored the indoor pool, more hot tubs, and the workout facility. By now it was time to get ready for lunch, which was held promptly at 11:15 a.m. The reason for this early time was that as people age, they go to bed earlier and thus get up earlier. If they're having breakfast at six in the morning, they're hungry by eleven. Wellington Hills had made the adjustment so they didn't have to.

"Susan, we need to see if the ice sculpture arrived."

I wanted to say, "What ice sculpture?! Are you kidding me?" But by now I knew to expect the unexpected. Or to put it differently, expect the opulent.

"What do you think?" Deborah said, as she opened up the freezer where an intricate buffalo had been carved from a block of ice. It looked massively time consuming—translation: expensive.

"It's fantastic. Do you have one every day?"

"Not every day. Maybe twice a week. Today's theme is Native American, so you'll see the menu is laid out accordingly."

I picked up a thick piece of parchment noting the date at the top. "Do you print up menus for each meal?"

"Yes, we do. We also have the same menu on the lower floor where all the other residents and visitors come. This second floor, though, has its own eating area due to the logistics, and each meal is planned in advance. Each menu also contains many of the residents' favorites, such as steak burgers and fries, mac and cheese, PB&J, and chocolate shakes. These are on every menu, because despite the hard work the chef puts in to the fancier offerings, sometimes a resident simply must go back to their roots.

I looked over the menu: Native American Catfish with Pine Nuts; Pinto Bean Bread with Prickly Pear Cactus Jelly; Chippewa Chicken Soup; Indian Fry Bread Tacos; Seminole Sautéed Alligator Tail; and Choctaw Pumpkin Cake. Setting it back down, I said, "You do this for each meal?"

"Yes. Well actually, Chef Andre does. He's a French-trained chef and is responsible for each meal. He and our dietician work out the menus weeks in advance so we can fly in the appropriate ingredients. I tasted the alligator yesterday; it's pretty good."

"Wow. So what do we do now?"

"Not much, really. Ms. Greenwald wants me to show you a typical meal here on the second floor. You will basically stand by in case there are problems or a resident needs something."

Deborah pointed to a spot where she wanted me to stand and greet the residents as they came in, *if* they appeared to want contact. Apparently some residents on the second floor occasionally had dark moods and refuse to make eye contact. It was up to me to figure that out.

It wasn't long before they started to arrive, with almost all of them being wheeled in. I introduced myself knowing none of them would remember my name. I smiled and greeted them warmly. When everyone was seated at their tables, I watched as each resident tried to focus on the menu and place their order. Many voices were raised and there were questions being asked over and over again. Suddenly, an elderly woman motioned for me. I took a couple steps towards her. "How can I be of service?"

Yelling as if I were across the room and not a mere foot away, she said, "Where are the *negroes* with my tea? I want my tea!"

Stunned, I replied, "Uhh . . . one moment, please. Let me get that for you."

Shaking her head, she turned away in disgust. I left for the kitchen, but Deborah intercepted me. "What did Mrs. Collier want?"

"She wants to know why her *negroes* haven't brought her tea."

Deborah chuckled. "Look, many of these residents grew up on wealthy ranches and had servants for everything. When dementia sets in they think they're back on the plantation. Our workers are used to it. Never mind her tea. One of the girls just brought it to her."

I looked around and saw that Mrs. Collier was now enjoying her tea, which had a fresh sprig of mint. Resuming my place, I continued to keep watch over the residents as they ate their food. Some engaged in conversation, while many others merely mumbled to themselves. A few sat in silence. Two of them lowered their faces to the table and fell asleep. Each time it happened a nurse sprang into action and either woke them up or wheeled them back to their room, making sure they didn't injure themselves. Overall, it was a very efficient process and a great learning experience, one that would surely be valuable wherever I ended up.

After my first week was over I arranged a celebration dinner with Vicki. She'd gotten the Granbury internship and was ready to compare notes. We met at a place called Riata's, a nice Texas-themed restaurant in downtown Fort Worth, and of course, we started out with wine.

"So Vicki, tell me about your experience in Granbury."

"Oh no you don't. You tell me yours first. I'm dying to find out what life's like for the rich and very rich."

"Okay," I said chuckling, "but I warn you, it's not going to be anything like your place."

She laughed. "I know that already."

"Alright, let me first tell you a bit about the place, then I'll tell you a story that happened today. First, each resident's monthly dues cover only one meal. They have to pay extra for additional meals, but that's not a problem because they all seem to have an endless supply of money."

"Wow! That *is* rich," she said, taking a sip of her Chardonnay.

"Yes, and occasionally a local doctor will come to the facility and perform minor outpatient surgery. How's that for a house call?"

"Not bad!"

"If the resident has to go to the doctor's office or the hospital, they go in either a Lexus, a Cadillac or a limousine, each supplying a man dressed like an old time chauffeur."

Vicki's eyes widened. "Man, that's going in style!"

I took a sip of my Shiraz. "The average age of each resident is eighty-four, with nobody under sixty. The oldest lady is 102. This last stat fits into my next story. Ready?"

"Sure. Let 'er rip."

"Today at lunch we had a nurse standing by a resident when out of nowhere, the resident barked at her. 'You go stand behind me. Servants should never be where you're standing. Know your place!' The nurse was Hispanic and she got very upset. She started telling me and the other nurses that she went to school, had to pass a test, has all the proper training and has never been called a servant. She's an LVN and it stung her hard."

"Yikes! These old folks take their prejudices with them wherever they go. I guess at that age they lose the ability to stop those thoughts from coming out."

I smirked. "That, or they choose not to stop them."

"Yeah, I guess you're right."

"Oh, and one more thing. Until recently, the nurses wore the old nurse outfits of white fitted stockings, white dresses, and a hat on top. Apparently, the residents were used to seeing that so they continued it way past the time the rest of society had moved on."

I continued with more stories about ice sculptures, alligator entrees, putting greens, and aviaries until I finally talked myself out.

"Boy, my stories aren't anything like yours. The closest thing in Granbury we have to an ice sculpture is when one of the residents dropped a large piece of ice that shattered into a million pieces. It did kinda look like art, though. And the only birds I've seen were when one man got mad because his chair was taken by another resident—he shot him the middle finger."

"Well, that doesn't sound too bad. You're probably learning more about nursing care and home skills than I am. Really, you are."

"Yeah, and on fish day we ran out of the cheap cod so the cook wadded up tiny pieces of chicken, dipped them in batter and they never knew the difference."

"That wouldn't happen at Wellington Hills. They'd never think of passing off one thing for another."

Vicki lowered her voice as her face grew serious. "I guess our cook had to take the alligator by the tail and solve the problem."

I started laughing again. "Yes, and that gator tail was tasty. Not saying I want it every day, but the way they prepared it was fantastic."

We shared some more laughs, drank our wine and ordered dinner. Afterwards, Vicki remembered something. "We do have something in common with Wellington Hills. We had a limo over the other day."

"Really, that's great!"

"No, it was taking away Mr. Jefferson. He'd died in his sleep."

"Oh," I said shaking my head. "That's terrible."

"Well, your place deals in reality, too. I mean, look how it's set up. As you get worse they lower you to the bottom floors so when you die you're that much closer to ground."

"True, or the loading bay."

"Death is the great equalizer, one the residents of Wellington Hills can't buy themselves out of."

"Yes," I said. "But they sure have a great time beforehand."

I'd been at Wellington Hills for two months when I finally got to see all that went into the preparation of each meal. Once in a while we were allowed to join the residents for lunch. Sitting at the table, I was able to fully appreciate the level of service, quality and detail that went into each meal. Elegantly folded cloth napkins were, of course, provided with plenty of spares since the residents dropped many of them on the floor—a floor that was kept immaculately clean. Each table had a thick, white linen tablecloth, above which rested the expensive china and silverware. The tablecloth had a dual function— it not only looked great but also provided enough texture to keep things from sliding off or spilling due to shaky hands or inadvertent elbows. Things still spilled, but it happened far less frequently with these nicer tablecloths. When a spill did occur, a staff member was there to wipe it up almost before the liquid hit the ground. It was an excellent, organized team.

After this particular lunch, I had to hustle to make sure one of the residents made it to the meeting room in the Burgundy hall. She wanted to meet with an interior designer and a fabric selection specialist to help pick out new curtains for her room. As soon as she had let us know she wanted them changed, we went to work scheduling in the right folks. It was amazing how easy things were to arrange when money was not a concern.

I had a number of duties each day. Sometimes I needed to meet with the wine supplier and ensure that the wine was put away properly. Other times I dealt with ice sculpture deliveries, bird feeder problems, or looking around the putting green for Mr. Penn's lost golf balls. Honestly, there was never a dull moment. Then there were the usual LNFA duties, such as resolving nursing issues with the Director of Nurses, ensuring residents were receiving adequate nutrition, checking on the maintenance of the building, training a launderer, keeping the budget in line, reviewing staff schedules and on and on. I was certainly learning a lot.

The next day after the lunch and fabric selections, we booked an opera singer for an impromptu performance. Most of the residents turned out, although I'm pretty sure a few turned off their hearing aids and began dozing. The singer didn't mind, especially with the check she was picking up.

That evening when my shift ended, I collected my purse and walked out to the employees' parking lot. I was just about to open my car door when a rough looking character came up to me.

"Say, you got some money to spare? I ain't eaten in days."

I was startled and unsure of how to respond. The employees' parking lot was open to the street and only a few blocks from a hangout for homeless people. This man appeared to be one of them. His hair was all matted, his clothes dirty and disheveled, and his demeanor was that of someone drunk or off his meds. I was still deciding what to do when out of nowhere, two policemen came storming over, took hold of the man, and forced him to the ground. Surprised, the man resisted, which caused one of the policemen to pepper spray his face. That ended the scuffle and shortly thereafter the man was handcuffed and tossed into a squad car, which arrived less than sixty seconds after the pepper spray had made its appearance. It was an unbelievably smooth operation, one that even SEAL Team Six could be proud of. After the squad car drove away, I turned to one of the police officers and said, "Boy, I'm sure glad you fellows were nearby. That guy was probably harmless, but you never know!"

The officer looked at me and said, "No problem, Ms. Hodges. That's our job. He was trespassing and had been warned many times in the past."

I was stunned and confused. "Wait, how do you know who I am? I never told you my name. Have we met before?"

"No, ma'am. Not really. We're off-duty police officers and work for Wellington Hills, just like you. We know everyone's car, where they park and their name. We kind of stay out of sight so we don't scare away any prospective residents. But we're always here, twenty-four seven, just out of sight. We also have other officers scattered around the place."

I nodded. "Yeah, I've seen them sometimes. I guess I just never put two and two together." I stared at the officer's gear. He had all the right equipment. This guy was no rent-a-cop. He was the real deal dressed in an actual police uniform. "Thanks again, officer. I really appreciate it."

He opened the door for me and said, "No problem, Ms. Hodges. Drive carefully."

Seeing him in my rearview mirror, I took off for home with yet another great story to tell Vicki.

❧

Finally, the full six months of my internship was over. One afternoon Ms. Greenwald called me into her office. "So Susan, did you learn a lot while you were here?"

"I sure did. A ton!" I wanted to tell her how much more I now knew about food, ice carvings, birds, fabric and armed security, but I was sure she already knew that stuff, too.

"Great, because I'm sending your paperwork to the state via over-night express and you should have your license in a week or so. I thought it was the least I could do for all the hard work you gave us. Also, here's an excellent reference," she said, sliding a letter over to me. "You may not find a place like this, but you should get a good chance at snagging one of the upper tier positions somewhere. If you need me to talk to someone, just let me know."

"Gosh, thanks so much! Not only for taking me on, but for all you've done for me. I won't forget it."

"I'm sure you won't, Susan, and do stay in touch with us. Let us know where you land. I'd love for you to get a great job and apply some of what you've learned here at another facility. Maybe you could even elevate the industry as a whole just a little bit more."

"I'll do my best, Ms. Greenwald."

We'd both stood up to say goodbye when she paused and added this, "Please don't forget what an LNFA is. She's the one who provides a safe and secure environment so the staff can perform their duties correctly. She's the one that ensures all residents who reside under her direction receive the highest quality of life and care possible. She's the one who maintains a resident's dignity and ensures all the residents' rights are upheld. She's the equivalent of a CEO who hires everyone and is responsible for everything. Even the owner can't tell her what to do. Just always do the right thing and take excellent care of the people that are placed in your hands. Their families, their loved ones and society in general are trusting you. Understand?

"Yes, ma'am. I sure do. That's great advice. I'll carry it with me wherever I go. Thanks again for everything."

We hugged and I walked out of Wellington Hills one last time before embarking on my own career as a licensed Texas LNFA. Now, it was time to find a ship to steer and a facility to run.

2

One month later, Vicki and I sat at the same table at the same restaurant. But now, things were different. "Gosh," Vicki said, "finding an LNFA position is gonna be harder than I thought. First, there's all the newly licensed administrators—let's say twenty of us in North Texas—who're competing with each other for the one or two available spots. Then there are the ones who've already been licensed for a while and have actual experience. We have to compete with them, too. There aren't enough jobs to go around."

I set my wine glass down. "No kidding! So I guess you and I have to make sure we get those two jobs, right?"

Vicki grinned. "I guess so, Miss Optimistic, though I'd sure like a chance to run Wellington Hills. That place sounded un-*freaking*-believable!"

I flashed back to the roasted pheasant I'd tasted on my last day, along with the intricate pheasant ice sculpture that sat in the middle of the dining room. "It sure was, but those places are even rarer than the two jobs currently available. Speaking of which, have you heard from either one of them?"

"Nah," she said, taking a sip from her wine glass. "All I got back from the Arlington one was an email saying they'd received my resume. The Dallas one hasn't replied yet. You?"

"Same thing. We'll just have to keep waiting and hoping. Maybe another one will pop up."

"Easy for you to say. I'm waiting to get married, and I think my boyfriend is planning on me supporting him while he stays home and plays video games all day. Without a job, it's unlikely we'll be getting married anytime soon."

"I know you're kidding. In fact, you're about my age when I was first married. And guess what? One day my second husband just up and died of a heart attack. Wham, bam and instantly I was unemployed with two kids to raise. I didn't have any type of career at that point. I daresay, you're not that bad off."

"Wow, Susan, I didn't know that. But it looks like you're doing well now."

"I don't know why you're saying that. I just spent a lot of money to become an LNFA and I'm still unemployed. You call that doing well?"

"I will if you'll pass the wine bottle."

We giggled and spent the rest of the night talking about subjects other than work, or the hunt for it. In other words—some girl time.

The next morning I stared at a number on my cell phone, one I didn't recognize. Touching 'Accept' I said, "Hello, this is Susan Hodges."

"Susan," a gruff voice came back. "I'm Billy Jones. I received your resume for an administrator's position and I'd . . ." (Loud coughing.) ". . . like to talk to you about it. Are you free today?" (More coughing.) Apparently, he was holding the phone away from his mouth.

I thought fast. I'd sent out resumes to several ads on the internet and in the newspaper, and had no idea which one this was. Sometimes the ads didn't even mention the name of the home. I assumed they probably still had an administrator in place and didn't want her to know. I ran through my schedule in my head and said, "Uh, yes. I'm available today."

"Okay, that's good. What about this morning, say 10 a.m.?"

Wow, this was sudden. "Uh, sure. Just give me the address to your office and I'll be there."

Again, more coughing. It sounded like he was dying. "I'm on the road right now. Can I meet you at the Chili's over on University?"

"That's fine, but are they open at ten in the morning?"

"Oh yeah, you're right. How 'bout 10:30?"

I wondered if this was a real deal. Do administrators get hired at Chili's? I decided to check it out anyway. I mean, what did I have to lose? "Okay, Mr. Jones. I'll be there. What do you look like?"

"First, just call me Billy. And second, I'll be standing next to a blue F-150 pickup, smoking a cigarette." This was followed by a loud hacking cough that sounded as if his left lung was coming up out of his throat.

"Yes, sir. I mean, Billy. See you then."

A click interrupted his nasty coughing spell. I stared at the phone and again wondered if this was a real call. Out of curiosity, I started looking through my applications, trying to figure out which one it was. None of them had anything with a Billy, William or Jones. Since it was only 8:30 a.m., I printed out a few more copies of my resume and began getting dressed.

The Chili's he picked was in a nice part of Fort Worth, very near Texas Christian University and the Colonial Golf Course—a regular stop for the PGA tour. The surrounding area held mostly expensive homes. I knew there were some nursing facilities nearby and hoped one of them needed an LNFA. That would be incredible. Could I be so fortunate as to land something like that?

I arrived a few minutes early and sure enough, there was a pudgy, gray-haired man slumped over the side of his F-150, smoking a cigarette. He wore jeans, a nice business shirt and well-worn brown shoes. I grabbed my portfolio and went to meet him. As I approached, I could see stains on his fingers from the cigarettes and a round stain on his front teeth. Clearly, he had a serious addiction. About twenty feet away, I said, "Are you Billy Jones?"

Exhaling a cloud of smoke, he said, "I sure am. You must be Susan Hodges."

"Yes," I said, smiling as we shook hands.

"Alright then, let's go inside and have a talk."

As we walked towards the entrance, he took as many puffs as possible before crushing out his cigarette in the large receptacle made for just that purpose. Exhaling his last cloud, he opened the door for me and we walked inside. I could tell they were barely ready for customers.

"Welcome to Chili's," a young girl said. "Would you like a table or a booth?" The girl sized up Billy and added, "Or perhaps you'd like to sit at the bar?"

Keeping silent, I waited during the awkward pause for him to decide. Was he seriously considering the bar?

"Well, let's go ahead and have a booth," he said finally.

As we followed the hostess, I began to appreciate the fact that we were in a public building. Again I thought, who meets in a Chili's to hire an administrator? And Billy looked like *he* needed a nursing home, not someone who worked for one. At this point I seriously doubted the man in front of me had anything to do with nursing homes or healthcare in general. This was probably a multi-level marketing opportunity, or a chance to become a straw buyer in an overappraised house and eventually go to prison.

"Here you are," she said, letting us slide in opposite of each other. "This is our lunch menu along with our drink specials. Your waitress is Celina and she'll be right with you. Thanks and enjoy."

Celina appeared just as Billy began eyeing the drink menu. "Hi, I'm your waitress. Can I get you folks some chips and queso to get started? Perhaps a frozen margarita?"

Billy looked at me and said, "What would you like, Ms. Hodges?"

"I'll have an iced tea, thank you."

Billy looked up at the waitress and said, "I'll have one, too. We're gonna talk for a bit while we're drinking our tea."

"Certainly," Celina said. "I'll be right back with your drinks."

When she'd disappeared, Billy started in. "I looked over your resume and I have a home I'm considering you for. This will be your first administrator's position, right?

"That's right," I said, nodding.

He moved the menus aside. "Okay, let me give you some background on the company. I'm the Director of Operations and my boss used to own over 250 nursing homes in Texas and Oklahoma. These were all fairly nice homes. Just over two years ago, he sold out to a large healthcare outfit in Denver. Part of his sales agreement restricted what he could do and where, but it didn't restrict him from buying low-level nursing homes. So he started buying 'em, fixing 'em up, and cash flowing 'em for a while, with the idea of building up a big pool of homes again and then selling out down the road. He hired me a while back and I basically run things. Now, I'm not trying to be ugly, but the truth is we're bottom feeders. These homes need work and have lots of challenges. Three months ago we purchased a field nursing facility nearby and I figured out the administrator was worthless. I need to hire someone to replace her." He started coughing and leaned into the aisle to do it. While he was bent over, things were starting to make sense to me. When he was done, he sat back up and continued. "Excuse me. Like I was saying, this gal was terrible and we'd been losing about $75,000 a month. Get the picture?"

"Yes," I said, just as the waitress brought our tea. "When do you need someone?"

"The day before yesterday," he said, shaking three sugar packets.

"So . . . right now?"

"Yes, right now!"

I took a deep breath and tried to weigh my options. Before I got too far, he jumped in and explained the salary and benefits, all of which were very good. We talked some more about the business and my past, and then he added this: "At all of our homes, we have a mission statement: God first, family second, and job third."

I certainly liked hearing that, as it matched my priorities. Maybe he wasn't such a rough character after all. I asked him, "Do you have any other candidates you're talking to?"

"Of course, and I'm not in the habit of making rash decisions. But right now my gut is screaming out to hire you!"

I raised my eyebrows and smiled. "Well Billy, I'm looking for a position as an administrator, so I'm available." I wondered if I was saying too much or not enough. Even though I knew I'd be good at whatever job I landed, I didn't want to blow this opportunity. So many nursing homes hired younger people with longer runways and, being in my late fifties with no experience, I needed to get my first job before I could get my second one.

"I'll tell you what, Susan. Let's drive over to the home right now and take a look, see what you think."

"Okay, I'll follow you."

Billy threw a twenty on the table and got up to leave. The hostess thanked us for coming and as soon as his hand was on the door, he flicked the Bic lighter and a trail of smoke drifted backwards into my face. Now we were both coughing.

After we got into our respective cars, Billy pulled his F-150 onto University and headed south. Surprisingly, he took a left and entered the 'no-fly' zone of Fort Worth. Every city has their war zones and Fort Worth is no different. Ours was called Red Nine. Back in the days when the train still ran through here, there was a stop called Red Nine and somehow the name stuck. Over time, this area had become the wasteland of Fort Worth. People saw the symbol of a nine as a dead person in a fetal position. The red stood for blood everywhere. It was rumored that the police in the Red Nine area stockpiled chalk and plastic yellow evidence tents at several locations for outlining bodies and marking the shells from drive-bys. According to legend, the police were always running out of both. In fact, funeral homes had hearses parked around the area on standby, just waiting to pick up dead bodies like tow trucks on busy highways hoping for broken-down vehicles. More than one person had suggested putting a tall fence around Red Nine and turning it into a maximum security prison with occasional airdrops of food, water and bullets. I was honestly hoping he was taking a short cut through the area. Unfortunately, he appeared to be headed for the dead center (with an emphasis on *dead*).

While we were stopped at a light, two local citizens came out of a store with 40-ounce adult beverages wrapped in brown paper. Since it was a little after 11 a.m., I told myself they must have just gotten off a late night shift and were winding down before they went to bed. Then I saw another gentlemen urinating on a bush next to two prostitutes. I couldn't really formulate a legitimate reason for why that was happening. Maybe he was dealing with a bladder problem? I wondered what the off-duty police officers at Wellington Hills would do about that.

Billy pulled in and parked in a handicapped space in a small asphalt lot on the side of an abandoned commercial building. A gust of smoke wafted out as he rolled down his window and stuck his arm out to signal for me to pull in next to him. As I did, I saw him reach down, grab a blue plastic handicapped permit and hang it on his rearview mirror. I met him at the back of his truck and started walking across the street to a decent looking building.

"Whoa Susan, where ya going?"

I stopped and turned around. "To check out your home. Isn't that why we're here?"

He chuckled. "Yeah, but that ain't our home. That's a commercial paper factory. This here's the home." He stuck his thumb out towards the abandoned building we had parked next to.

Confused, I stared at the building and began to worry about this little trip. "Uhh, I thought you said it was up and running with an administrator you recently fired."

Billy pulled the lit cigarette out of his mouth, exhaled politely away from me, and stepped closer. "Okay, here's the deal Susan. When folks run out of their money before they run out of life, this is where they end up. The feds and the state pay Medicaid, Medicare—whatever we can collect for these poor folks to stay in places like this. This is the last stop for them. Most of these folks had good quality lives before, but misjudged their savings or insurance company limits. Instead of letting 'em die on the streets, the government pays for them to live in places like these."

In school, I had studied facilities like the ones he just described, but I hadn't seen one up close. Because our healthcare system was keeping people alive longer than ever before, more and more people were running out of resources and had nowhere else to go. Of course, I never thought I'd actually be running one. "So, you're saying people are in there right now?"

"Yeah, about eighty."

"In that building right there?" I pointed to it to make sure there was no miscommunication.

"Yes, that one!" he said, obviously irked.

"With no staff? Come on!"

Billy put his hands on his hips. "Why do say that?"

I pointed at the parking spaces. "Look, we're the only two cars here and there's only room for four more. If you had staff, this lot would be overflowing."

Frustrated, he puffed harder on his cigarette. Suddenly, I got nervous about the prospect of walking into an abandoned building with someone I'd just met. I had no proof he was a Director of Operations or that he even had a job available. This was heading south fast.

Billy finished his cigarette, dropped the butt on the ground, and crushed it out with his scuffed brown shoe. Then he looked me directly in the eyes. "Susan, there's probably thirty staff in there right now. I need you to understand, the people who work here are poor too. They don't have money for a car. They all take the bus. And any visitors the residents have—which is rare—also take the bus. This is a poor place for poor people and it's located in a poor area. Right now I need an administrator, someone to turn it into something good and turn a profit. Sure, it's gonna be hard work. But you also need your first job. We both need something here. Now, why don't we go in, take a look, and see what you think. I need to hire someone as an admin for this home and right now that person is you."

I stood there undecided. It was possible I could wait it out for a better opportunity, but I had no idea how long that would be. I wasn't getting any younger and I was here. At least I could go in. "Okay, let's take a look."

Billy nodded and said nothing as he led me to the entrance. Now I could see that there were people inside and knew it wasn't abandoned, although it sure seemed like it needed to be. Everywhere there was worn equipment, worn furniture, worn staff and worn residents. Everyone and everything was worn, with a few items looking worn *out*. The absolute nicest word I could think of to describe this place was 'pitiful.'

"What's it called?" I said.

"The Jones-Simms Nursing Center."

"I assume you're the Jones, but who's the Simms?"

Billy looked around to make sure no one was listening, then lowered his voice. "Jones and Simms were famous high school athletes from this area, so we were hoping to capitalize on their names. You know, sort of a brand recognition kind of thing. Really, there's no Simms. It's just a coincidence it matches my last name."

I hated deception, but I continued on. When we completed the tour, I noticed he hadn't introduced me to any of the staff and none of them had introduced themselves to me. In fact, most of them avoided eye contact. That seemed odd.

Billy led me to a small closet and closed the door for privacy. "Okay Susan, you've seen the place. I like your resume. You seem levelheaded. You don't seem like a quitter. You probably don't mind hard work. As you can see, this is one fine challenge. The last admin wasn't up to the task. What do you say? Want the job?"

I thought for a few seconds and knew this might be my only chance for a long while. I was just going to have to make the best of it. "Yes Billy, I'll be your admin. When do you want me to start?"

He looked at his watch. "It's almost noon. If you start now I'll pay you for the whole day."

I blinked several times. "Okay, I guess I'll have to start sometime. Might as well be now. Just take me to my office. I get claustrophobic in small closets."

Billy rubbed his jaw and stuck out his hand. "Susan, you're officially hired right? You're not going to quit on me?"

I shook his hand. "No Billy, I'm not a quitter. I'll get the job done . . . *somehow.*"

"Good. I'll have one of the girls call you and get your payroll info. By the way, this here's your office." With that he turned and left the building.

3

I walked into the main hallway and took a look around. One resident was pushing himself down the corridor in an old, beat-up wheelchair. Drool was dripping onto his shirt and he seemed oblivious to his surroundings. Another resident sat in a chair, her right arm shaking as she stared at the wall. A young Hispanic man in overalls carrying a pipe wrench appeared from one room and was about to enter another when I called out to him. "Sir, excuse me, do you work here?"

The man stopped. "Yes, do you need something?"

I approached him and put out my hand. "Hi, I'm Susan Hodges. I'm your new administrator. I was just hired by Billy Jones."

His eyes narrowed and focused for a moment before flying wide open. "Oh, okay!" he said, shaking my hand and smiling. "I'm Carlos Cortez, the Maintenance Director."

"Pleased to meet you, Carlos. So how many staff do you supervise?"

"Staff? Please, it's just me. I'm the director and the workers all rolled into one."

This was a change. At Wellington Hills we had four workers supervised by a maintenance director and an assistant maintenance director. "Okay. Have you seen the business office manager?"

"I think she's gone."

I glanced at my watch and saw it was close to lunchtime. "Okay. Do you have a moment to show me around? That is, unless you're in the middle of something."

"It can wait. Let's go."

Still carrying his wrench, he led me on a tour down each hall. While we walked, I learned he'd been at the home for six months and was retained by Billy when they bought the place three months ago. Carlos told me he was doing his best with what little he had to work with. He pointed to the walls, which had been repainted with the original colors from the late sixties and early seventies—avocado, orange, and dark brown. The paint itself looked half an inch thick, as if each painter had simply slapped on a new coat over the old stuff. Then he pointed out the flooring. Where there was carpet, its original dark brown color was now black with stains and worn through to the concrete in some places. The pattern on the vinyl floor tile was almost gone too. Even though the building was only one story, it seemed to go on forever. After I'd seen most of the common area, I was surer than ever that the building needed to be demolished. I could see Carlos had a huge challenge keeping everything up and running.

When we got to the kitchen, Carlos introduced me to the Food Services Director, Alisha Pogue, and then left us to talk. Her staff had served lunch at 10:30 a.m. and was in the process of cleaning up.

"Alisha, how many staff do you supervise?"

"Three, when they all show up. I prepare most of the food myself, and if I'm lucky, they're around to help. Then we clean up and begin on the next meal."

Looking around, I saw that most of the wooden cabinets that held all the dishes and various ingredients were coming loose from the walls with several close to falling. Also, the lacquer sealer was long gone. Pointing to a cabinet, I said, "How do you clean these?"

She frowned. "You really can't. The wood warps and rots if you spray anything on it. We try to wipe them down with a damp cloth, but that's all we can really do."

I looked at the fryer. The sides were black with years of grease build-up. "Can you clean this off?"

Her frown deepened. "We've scrubbed and scrubbed, but it's so baked on we can't make a dent."

I shook my head. This would be a real problem during health inspections. Yet I could see the grease had been there for years, if not decades. Somehow it had passed before, though I had no idea how.

"Could you please show me the dining room?"

Alisha led me to an open area dotted with chipped tables and dented wooden chairs—several with the arms broken off. The fabric on many of the seats was torn and in some cases worn through to the supports below. Seeing my shock, Alisha walked over to the large bay window. "They can all look out this window while they eat."

I went up and looked out myself. There I saw a small area open to the sky and enclosed with four brick walls, much like a prison yard. It was mostly dirt with a few patches of grass and weeds. Positioned in two locations were large cooking pans, black from use as ashtrays. For some reason cigarette butts were scattered everywhere around them, as if moving another twelve inches to hit the pans would've been too much effort. There was also a concrete patio with a few pieces of plastic furniture.

When I turned back around to talk to Alisha, she was speaking with one of her workers. I realized that not only was she very busy, but I hadn't eaten lunch. "Alisha, I'm going to let you get back to work. I'll finish my tour with some of the other folks."

She nodded and left me alone in the empty dining room. What I'd seen so far was completely pathetic—worse than I'd imagined after talking to Billy. When my stomach grumbled for the third time I decided to leave and get a bite, or at least try to find some place safe to eat.

After navigating my way out of the Red Nine area, I found a sandwich shop and downed a sub. I dialed Vicki when I got back to my car.

"Hey, Susan," she said, answering the phone. "What's up?"

"I just got a job!"

"What?!" she said in disbelief. "As an admin?"

"Yes, as an admin. It's crazy! The Director of Ops called this morning and asked if we could meet. He hired me on the spot. Since he wanted me to start right away, I'm working at the home today. I just took a break to grab some lunch."

"Now I know you're kidding. Nobody hires anyone that fast. They have to do background checks and drug tests. There's no way."

"There *is* a way. They fired the administrator and needed someone right now, and that someone is me."

"I'm stunned! And I'm so jealous. But of course, I'm also happy for you. What's the name of the home?"

"The Jones-Simms Nursing Center."

Silence.

"Vicki, are you still there?"

"Yes." A long pause. "You're teasing me, right?"

"No. As I said, I'm working there right now. What's the matter?"

Vicki paused yet again. "A few days ago Michele—you know, from class—was called to interview there and talked to our placement director, Ms. Hightower. She found out some guy was calling all the newly licensed LNFAs and setting up meetings at the nursing home, but the women drove off before he could interview them. So he started meeting them at restaurants, discussing salary and benefits first before showing them the place. It's supposed to be a real hellhole. But . . . I guess you work there now so it's, ah . . . real nice?"

"Well, the truth is, it's in a bad location, and yes, it's pretty run-down. But I decided to take the job anyway. I need the income. Hopefully it'll be safe."

Vicki softened her tone. "I'm sure it's great. I mean, I guess I'm happy for you. At least now I don't have to compete against you for a job, right?"

"Yes," I said sarcastically. "That's right. So that's good news for you."

"And if something bad happens to you, there'll be another job opening, so that'll take away another competitor. So hey, things are pretty good then." Now I knew Vicki was just being Vicki. Before I could respond, she added, "I think you'll do well. Really, if anyone can turn-around . . . *something like that* . . . it's you!" Finally, some sincerity.

"Thanks. I appreciate that. But listen, I have to get back to work before they start thinking I drove off and am not coming back, okay?"

"Sure, and Susan, please be safe, okay? That place is in Red Nine, right?"

"Yes it is, and I will. Don't worry. I'll call you tonight so I can hear some more sarcasm."

I hung up and drove back to the home, somewhat upset. First, because she acted like I was stupid for taking the job. Second, because Billy had been running through applicants and I was simply the next warm body to plug in. That attitude came back with me when I arrived at the parking lot and again, had a complete selection of spaces. When I locked my car, I saw several men loitering in the area and wondered how safe my car would actually be. Would it still be there when the workday was over? Who knows?

The moment I walked inside the front door a woman in nursing scrubs confronted me. She was holding adult diapers in both hands. "Are you the new admin?"

"Yes, I'm Susan Hodges. Can I help you?"

"I'm Regina Johnson, Director of Nursing. We've got a problem." She looked very flustered. Several residents were in the area milling around and I didn't want them being bothered with our problems so I walked with her to my closet-for-an-office. "I'd ask you sit down, but apparently I don't have any chairs."

"That's because the business office manager took them along with your desk and moved it all into her office down the hall. She was using a small foldout table and replaced it with your stuff—or the last admin's stuff."

"I see. By the way, where is my BOM?"

"She's gone."

"That's the second time I've heard that. Where did she go?"

Regina rolled her eyes upwards. "Umm, I think to Warm Heart, but I may be wrong."

"What's Warm Heart?"

Pointing in the direction of the courtyard, she said, "It's the nursing home behind us. There are several in the area and everyone basically swaps employees all the time. I came from Colonial Hills. And Carlos, the maintenance director, came from Skyline Care."

I realized she was telling me my business office manager had quit, but set that aside to discuss her urgent problem. "Okay, let's get back to your situation. What exactly is it?"

She thrust the incontinent diapers at me. "*This* is our problem. Today's Wednesday and we won't receive a new order of diapers until Friday. We're not gonna make it. The two new residents are going through them like Billy goes through cigarettes."

The visual image almost made me laugh. "Alright. What can we do to make them last?" I knew she was holding the professional version which was very expensive. We were probably on a periodic delivery. I could call the company and increase the order, but unless I pulled out my own credit card and bought the cheaper consumer kind, we'd have to make do.

"Well, I was hoping you had some ideas."

I remembered something we did at Wellington Hills when a resident had a bad rash. "Can we leave them off at night and let their skin air out?"

"Sure, I guess. That might actually help some of them. They get bad rashes and could use a break. We can open up a diaper and keep it under them while they sleep. Most of them don't roll around in bed so we should be okay."

"Great! Now during the day can we make a portable potty chair available to the ones who are in better shape?"

"Sure, we can do that. We have four of them, but they're missing rollers, slide sideways and squeak badly. One has a crack that could use duct tape."

I thought for a moment. "Alright, go find Carlos right now and tell him to take the squeaks out with some WD-40, tape up the one chair as best he can, and see if he can make adjustments to keep them from going sideways. Also, let's get the mops out and ready to go for any resident that has an accident. And if a diaper is still in good shape, see if we can keep 'em on a few hours more. When you get all that handled, bring me a count of how many diapers you think we'll need and I'll call and increase the order. Okay?"

Regina seemed calmer. "Yeah, that should work. Actually, I guess it'll have to work."

"That's right. Now I'm going to try to find my desk and chairs and get this place set up."

Regina left with a better attitude. I knew from my experience in other industries that some people liked building up problems into something worse just in order to cause chaos. Others enjoyed getting worked up. I wasn't sure yet if Regina was either one of these, but I was going to keep an eye on her.

I started walking around the facility and visiting with the residents. I was shocked at their age. At Wellington, there was barely anyone under eighty. Here, we had lots of residents in their fifties and sixties and even one in his forties. Sure, we still had the seventies and eighties, but it was completely skewed twenty years younger than Wellington Hills.

As I made my way around, I introduced myself to the rest of the staff. The staff was fairly thin—with many of the positions filled simply to comply with the minimum legal requirements. I came upon Carlos working on the potty chairs. He was able to take some of the squeak out and fix most of the problems, but not the sideways rolling. If it rolled sideways when a resident went to sit down, it could cause a fall. Falls to elderly people were often fatal. If not immediately, then soon afterwards. That was a big concern.

When Carlos was done I had him help me move the desk and two chairs back into my tiny office. I was just arranging things when Dona Yancey, our Social Services Director, came bursting into my office.

"Susan, we've got a problem."

I looked up from trying to wipe my desk clean. "Okay, sit down and tell me about it." I was getting used to these "we've got a problem" statements.

Dona was too excited to sit down, so instead she launched into a description of the current disaster. This one involved a female resident, Betsy, who was in her late seventies. Betsy Dowell had a son in his fifties and according to Dona, he was a drug addict. He would come to the home, check Betsy out, take her on the street and prostitute her out for drug money. The past administrator had either been too scared to say no, or simply didn't care. Either way, he was back and looking for the administrator, the one who'd been fired.

When Dona told me this story, I calmed her down and said I'd handle it. I got up from my desk and walked to the lobby where he stood waiting. I was certain Dona had the story all wrong, so I decided to hear his side of the story.

"Hi there. I'm Susan Hodges. How can I help you?"

"I'm takin' my momma out of here. Are you gonna go get her or do I have to do it myself?"

I looked the man over. He was shaking, sweating and appeared to have been sleeping in a dumpster for quite some time. I was beginning to believe the drug part.

Trying to keep the man calm, I said, "Well, I'm new here. Why don't you come back in a few days after I've had some time to go over your mother's file. Let me see what her medical needs are and I'll assess the situation. If everything's good, she can leave." I was on shaky ground here because legally the resident could leave for short periods of time if they were of sound mind. Yet I didn't have any idea if she was. The moment I told him, however, his demeanor changed.

Pointing and raising his voice, he barked, "Look bitch! My momma needs to work the streets. Are you gonna go get her or do I need to?"

I held my hands up. "No problem, sir. It's just that I have to note in her file where she's going. When you say 'work the street,' what do you mean? You know, so I can add it to her file."

He took a step towards me. "Work the streets! Turn some tricks! You know, for some *johns*? Now go get her. She wants to go with me, so don't make me get hopped in here 'cuz you ain't gonna like it!"

Keeping my hands up I said, "Yes, sir. Let me get her ready. Just calm down. We don't want any trouble."

I turned to Dona, "Come with me." When we were out of his hearing, I said, "Go get Carlos and that boy in food services. Tell them what's going on and to find a reason to hang around the lobby."

She ran off to get them while I walked swiftly to his mother's room, which she shared with another woman. I knocked on the door. "Who is Mrs. Dowell?"

A frail lady in the far bed said, "I am."

I walked over and drew the curtain, separating us from the other resident. "Mrs. Dowell, I'm the new administrator, Susan Hodges. Listen, your son is here and wants to take you out." Upon hearing those words she got out of bed and began putting on her clothes. I stopped her. "Ma'am, do you know where he's taking you?"

"Yes," she nodded. "He's taking me out to his neighborhood."

"Yes, but do you know why?" I feared her answer.

"He wants to sell me so he can get money for drugs."

That confirmed it. I wanted to throw up just thinking about some man actually paying money to have sex with her. It was pure evil. "Ma'am, do you know what you're saying?"

She stared at me for a few seconds before speaking. "I know my son's a drug addict. He's been a drug addict for many years. And yes, I prostitute myself out to help him."

I was completely floored. By this time, my director of nursing was standing at the doorway. "Regina," I whispered, "act like you're helping get her ready, but delay things. I'm calling the police." She nodded and went to help Mrs. Dowell.

Moving fast, I returned to the lobby where I saw Carlos and the food service boy stationed near Mr. Dopehead. "Sir, they're getting her ready. I need to get a form for you to sign because you're going to be responsible for her. Do you understand?"

"Yeah, whatever. Just make it quick."

I ran to my office, jerked up the receiver and called 9-1-1. The operator was having a hard time believing me once I explained the situation, but went ahead and dispatched the officers anyway. With them on the way, I found a generic form, grabbed a pen and walked slowly back to the lobby.

"Sir, would you come over here and help me fill this out?"

He came grudgingly. I pulled out a chair for him so when he sat down his back would be to the police. Then, in excruciating detail, I began filling in the form with useless information. I asked for his full name and address. I had him give me the purpose for taking her out and the street she'd be working. I got his social security number, which I was surprised he gave me. He even gave me his cell phone number. I just kept going and going until I ran out of items. He made no fuss, thankfully, despite my ridiculous questions. Then I had him sign it. The second he set the pen down I looked over his shoulder and saw two Fort Worth police officers coming in through the front door. Their hands were on their weapons. Seeing me with Mr. Dopehead, they spread out in case the man was armed.

"What seems to be the problem here?" the lead officer said.

Hearing their voices, the man spun his head around fast and saw the two officers. He turned back to me and yelled, "You bitch! I'll get you for this!" He pointed at my staff. "All of you bitches are dead too!"

I jumped away from him and said, "This man wants to prostitute out his seventy-four-year-old mother for drug money. I even had him sign this form stating which streets she'd be working."

When Mr. Dopehead heard that, his eyes darted furtively to alternate exits. He looked like he was about to bolt. Seeing this, one officer yelled, "Stand up, sir! And get your hands up. Grab some wall. Now!"

The man stood up slowly, keeping his arms by his sides. He was sizing up the officers. That was the moment I realized this was about to get crazy. Instantly, we all scattered. As I ran away, the last thing I saw was the officers unsnapping their guns. I learned later that when he heard the unsnapping, he decided to go ahead and grab some wall. They got the handcuffs on and escorted him to a patrol car. A third officer came in and took down our information. Looking at the form he'd signed, which was basically a full confession, the officer laughed. "We'll be calling you later to get more information, but with this guy's outstanding warrants, chances are his mother will have passed away by the time he gets out of prison."

I followed him outside and watched them drive away with this criminal squirming around in the back. I was thrilled he'd be locked up. When I came back inside, my entire staff was clapping. I had just passed my first big test. That's when I knew I had a chance to last at this job.

Five months later his mother passed away while Mr. Dopehead was serving a four-year prison term. Thankfully, nobody was ever harmed . . . *yet*.

4

When my first Monday rolled around I pulled up to the facility and parked in my usual spot. Mornings were the only pleasant time in Red Nine since most of its citizens were sleeping it off and wouldn't be up until 11:00 a.m. at the earliest. As a result, I felt safest in the mornings. That all changed by the time I was ready to leave at the end of the day, when I was more than worried as I made the short walk to my car. Even the drive out of Red Nine kept me on edge.

The nature of the neighborhood caused me to value our special side entrance. Painted to blend in with the brick exterior, a single metal door directly faced the parking lot. Each morning I got out of my car in a hurry, walked briskly to the door with the correct key in hand, and made a super speedy entrance. Once inside, I closed the door quickly and locked the two dead bolts. It was only then that I felt I could relax. At quitting time I'd look out the peephole, see if the coast was clear and then make a dash for it. Maybe I was making more out if it than necessary, but then again, maybe not. There certainly were no Wellington Hills police officers around to save me.

Yet this morning I decided to do something different—I stopped, lowered my head, put my right hand on the door and said a prayer for the residents and the staff. I asked God to help me treat all the residents with respect and dignity and treat the staff with kindness and understanding. Then I unlocked the door and went inside. Somehow, I felt better.

My first task was to call the director of nursing into my office. I wanted to get down to business right away.

"How are we doing with the incontinent diapers?"

"Fine," Regina said. "The supply we received late Friday will tide us over until the next delivery. With the increase you called in, we should be okay."

"Okay, good. But each time we add a resident, let's assess their needs and coordinate an increase, if need be."

Regina nodded. "Great idea."

"Next, I've been studying these residents' health charts and frankly, I'm not sure what to make of them. It appears that at least 80% are addicted to alcohol or had alcoholic relatives and 85% were smokers. Is that right?"

"Yes, that's right. Many of them still smoke. That's why we have all those ashtrays out in the courtyard. But forget the alcohol and cigarettes. Have you counted the ones with gunshot or stab wounds? And the drug use! My Lord, it's amazing many of them are still alive!"

I shook my head in disbelief. "Yes, you're right. Do these folks have any visitors?"

"Most don't. There might be an occasional family member or friend. But really, the only friends they have are each other, the ones inside this home. That's it."

"That's pretty sad. They look highly depressed, not lively at all. What can we do to improve things?" Raised voices suddenly echoed outside my office, interrupting our meeting. "What's going on?"

We followed the sounds to the dining room where we saw a commotion in the courtyard. Several residents were raising their fists and pointing at the fence. I hustled outside to find Dona, the social services director, trying to calm everyone down. "What's going on?" I asked.

Dona threw her hands up in the air. "Oh, another scrap with Warm Heart. Sometimes our residents get into it with their residents. Usually it's just a lot of shouting and shooting the bird at each other." I moved past her and approached the low fence. "Be careful, Susan," she yelled. "Sometimes they throw things."

I looked cautiously over the dilapidated wooden boards and saw a large backyard area similar to our own. There were perhaps ten residents standing around smoking cigarettes, all staring at me. One of them shouted out, "Your home sucks!" Then I saw two older men standing together, about twenty feet away from the fence. One of them had a full head of jet-black hair and the other bright red. They seemed strangely odd.

"Excuse me," I said. "I'm the new administer here. Do you folks have a problem? Perhaps I could . . ."

The red haired man extended his middle finger. "~~Fuck you!~~ Warm Heart is better than your ~~fucking~~ shelter!"

My jaw dropped. Before I could reply, the man with black hair shouted, "Go back to your dump!" Then he shot me the bird too. Many of the other residents joined in, giving me the one-finger salute. I blinked a few times to make sure of what I was seeing. All I could manage was a "Have a blessed day," before turning around and hustling back to the patio, hoping they didn't throw anything.

When I was out of range, I said to both Regina and Dona, "Why do they hate our place so much?"

Regina moved closer and lowered her voice. "Because our residents give it right back to them. It's kind of a rivalry thing. You know, 'My nursing home's better than yours.' That kind of thing."

I shook my head. "So our residents do it right back? I can't believe this."

"Believe it," said Dona. "It makes our residents happier to think someone else has it worse. The same goes for the residents at Warm Heart. In fact, our residents call them Heart Worm. It's really crazy."

"There were two characters, one with black hair and the other with red hair. What are they all about?"

Regina laughed. "We call 'em Red Man and Old Blackie. The one with black hair has a toupee while Red Man apparently dyes his hair. With Kendra there now, I'm sure they're stirred up plenty."

"Kendra? Our former business office manager?"

"Yeah, she went over there the day you showed up. She was hoping to get the administrator's position."

"Does she have a license?"

They both chuckled. "No, but before the new company bought us that didn't matter much."

"That reminds me," I said, "I'd better get back inside and start looking for a BOM. It seems like things have calmed down for now. Call me if it flares up again."

As I walked away Dona said, "We will. And don't worry, it will."

A few hours later I had an employment ad placed and turned my attention to the facility itself. According to the state, Jones-Simms was certified for 115 beds. But because the company had turned some of the rooms into offices, we could only hold 96 residents. At present we had only 71. Since most people here were on Medicaid, just about everyone had to share a room. If a resident wanted a private one, they'd have to find somebody to pay the difference. Also, the money couldn't be in the resident's name, because the state only allowed a person to have $2,000 in cash and assets to receive Medicaid. The state of Texas also mandates that a resident have a minimum of 80 sq. ft., even though the cells on death row are 86 sq. ft. Each room has its own bathroom, which the two residents share, and a pull curtain separates the two sides of the room (like the ones in emergency rooms). They have a small dresser, a bed and a tiny closet with a rack for only a few items. It's very small and very sad.

As I learned more about the law for residents living at this level, I had to keep telling myself that this was the way it was. If I wanted to make a difference, I had to do my best with what I had. So that's what I set to doing.

A few hours later Dona knocked on my door. "Susan, we have a resident coming back to the home. You ought to check this out."

"I'll be right there," I said, grabbing a pen and paper. I then made my way to the main entrance where an ambulance was unloading a woman onto a gurney and wheeling her in. Regina was already there with a CNA (certified nursing assistant) waiting to take over.

They held the door open for the attendants, one of whom asked, "Where do you want her?"

Regina pointed down the hall. "Follow the CNA. The room is there on the left." The gurney rolled to an empty room. "Put her in the bed closest to the door. That way, it'll be easier to keep an eye on her."

The attendants unloaded the resident and handed me a clipboard. Looking at it I said, "What do you want from me?"

"Your signature," he said indignantly. "She's your resident."

"She is? That's news to me." I had a complete list of our residents and she wasn't one of them.

Regina grabbed the clipboard, signed the form and sent the men on their way. "Give me a second, Susan. I'll be in your office to explain. I just need to check her out." With that she turned her attention back to the resident and barked out orders to her assistant and another CNA who'd just arrived.

Fifteen minutes later, Regina was in my office plopping down in the chair and sighing. "Okay, let me fill you in on Lucy. She's our resident pole dancer."

"Pole dancer?!" This job was getting crazier by the moment.

"Yeah, she used to be a pole dancer—or an exotic dancer as they call them now."

"You mean a stripper?"

"Sure. She did that for most of her life, until she ended up here. The problem is, she doesn't seem to have ever had a home. She feels like this is a motel or something temporary so occasionally, she runs away. We try to tell her it's her home and that she belongs here, but the lure of the streets is too much. The police usually find her pretty quickly and bring her back. This time, though, she was gone for a full three weeks, so we boxed up her stuff—which wasn't much—and stored it in the shed. Well, they found her in some abandoned house that was condemned and barely standing. She was sleeping on a nasty old mattress for weeks. It's crazy.

"That's terrible!" I said. "How is she now?"

Regina shook her head. "Not good. She was taken to the hospital and treated for an infection and scabies. Since she's indigent, they did an S & S—a stabilize and ship. We're the lucky recipients. But at least we can resume payment from the state, so it's not all bad."

"Oh boy, I learn something new here every day."

She chuckled. "Get used to it. This is the way it is."

"Alright, since I don't have a BOM, I guess I'll get on the paperwork myself. Someone's gotta make sure we get paid so we can make payroll."

Regina stood up to leave, and then turned back to me. "Oh, she's got a bad infection and might not make it. They found her pretty frail and malnourished. We'll do what we can, but you might want to get on the paperwork as quickly as possible. If she dies before you get it in, the state has a way of not paying. I'd overnight it if I were you."

"Gee, that's nice of them. Thanks for the heads up. I'm sure you'll do what you can to save her, if it's possible."

"Sure," she said, before closing my door behind her.

I picked up Lucy's police and medical records and began preparing the report.

It was almost quitting time when the phone rang. Since the receptionist wasn't answering, I picked it up. "Jones-Simms Nursing Center, Susan Hodges speaking. May I help you?"

"You haven't quit yet?" It was Billy Jones.

"No, not yet. Though it's sure an adventure."

"That's the nicest word I've heard for it." His laugh morphed into a hacking cough.

"I haven't been here a full week and already I've had a dope head threaten our lives, been cussed out by the residents in the nursing home behind us, and witnessed a runaway brought back on a gurney. Add to that surviving a shortage of incontinent diapers and one could say I've stretched my talent to its limits."

He started laughing/coughing again. "Well, I think I hired the right person!"

I decided not to mention the fact that I was the first applicant who actually went inside the building. "Since you're so happy, Billy, I have to ask for something."

"Uh oh, hang on. Let me get a hold of my wallet."

"Why don't you pull it out and look inside it, because this facility is almost ready to be demolished. We need to fix some things around here and I have some ideas." I knew I was being bold, but I was hoping he might listen.

"Susan, we're losing $75,000 a month. It's not like we have extra cash. Besides, I'm constantly working on getting you more residents so we can one day turn a profit. We can think about fixing a few things then."

"Come on, Billy. I know when you buy these rundown places you expect to put in some money and fix them up. Right? That's how you flip them."

"I plead the fifth," he said, skipping the laughter and going straight to the coughing.

"Well, I have some ideas and I'd like to tell you about them, see what you think."

Silence.

"Billy?"

Finally he said, "Okay, let's have it."

I spent the next thirty minutes laying out my plan of action, one I hoped would be affordable to the company while showing the staff and residents we were improving their lives. When I finished, Billy said he'd discuss it with the owner and get back to me. It was the best I could hope for.

By Friday, I had several serious applicants for the business office manager position, one of whom was Melva Wooten. Seated before me was a polite, nicely dressed woman who had years of experience as an administrator. I thought she would be an excellent hire, yet I wanted to make sure.

"Tell me Melva, why do you want to step down to a business office manager, especially when you have a license to make more money as an administrator?"

"That's a fair question," she said calmly. "And I have a truthful answer. I was an administrator at my last job for nine years, but starting my fourth year, something happened, something very bad. I was sitting at my desk one day—much like you are right now—when this man came in and showed me some fancy ID. He was from the IRS. He asked, 'Are you Melva Wooten?' I said, 'Yes, what can I do for you?' He sat down and said, 'Melva, you owe the IRS $4.9 million.' I said, 'What? I don't even make over $150,000 a year. How could I owe you that much? This has to be a joke, right?' He said, 'Oh no, it's no joke.' Then he put his briefcase on my desk and pulled out dozens of deposit slips. 'Is this your signature here?' I told him, 'Yes.' He said, 'Did you sign the back of these checks?' I said, 'Yes, why?' Then he dropped the hammer. 'When you signed your name it made you responsible for the taxes that were never paid.' Well, my heart sure started racing, let me tell you! Then he went on and showed me all the accounts I'd opened up for the owner since he lived in another state. I'd been sending the owner money each month and he'd never paid the FICA, the unemployment tax or any of the money we withheld. He'd kept it all. When I explained that I could sell everything I owned and still not come up with $4.9 million, the IRS agent didn't care. Once I stopped panicking we were able to come up with a plan. To begin with, each month I had to start keeping the withholding in an account the owner couldn't touch. This kept me from digging a deeper hole. Then I started secretly siphoning off some additional money to pay the back taxes. It took me over six years of slowly making payments, but I did finally get it all paid off. On that day, a different man from the IRS came out and gave me a document showing I was cleared of any wrongdoing. With that in hand I emailed my notice to the owner and decided never to be an administrator again. I took a few months off to celebrate my freedom and now I'm back looking for work as a business office manager. Frankly, you can have all the administrator work you want."

I leaned back and swallowed hard. That was truly a frightening story, one that made me wonder if I could get into a trap like that with Billy. I put the thought aside and spent the next hour asking her more questions before deciding to hire her, pending a check of her references. We shook hands and she left. Once all of the references checked out, I called her back and offered her the job. She happily accepted and agreed to start the upcoming Monday.

With that problem solved, I decided to call a staff meeting. Of course, we had no conference room—the best we could do was set up space in the dining room and put the CNAs on guard duty to steer away any curious residents. When everyone was assembled, I stood and addressed the management staff. "As you folks know, I want to begin improving things around here, but we have next to no money. Still, I have approval from management to spend a little here and there, so I've started thinking of all the areas that need the most help. First, there's nursing. The nurses have terrible lockers in the dressing area. They all need upgrading and the scheduled drug locker also needs some work." I saw Regina and her assistant DON nodding their heads.

"The facility itself could use so much work it's hard to know where to start." This time Carlos nodded his head. "And the residents' rooms need to be completely redone, including the bathrooms. But with the small budget I've received, I decided it's best to begin with an area that affects both the staff and the residents, and with some luck, maybe we can make things a whole lot happier. That area is food services." At this, Alisha's face lit up and she silently clapped her hands.

"Food is served three times a day and even the staff occasionally has something to eat. Plus, the residents' moods are greatly affected by their meals. That's why I'm going to slowly rebuild the food prep area first. We can tackle the other, much more challenging areas afterwards. The first item I have approval to replace are the cabinets since they're literally falling off the walls and pose a safety risk. I also have enough money to replace the countertops. This will take a good chunk of money, but I feel that giving our food prep people better working conditions will allow them to start preparing better meals and perhaps add a dose of love into them. Thoughts?"

A lively discussion ensued which eventually validated my plan. Everyone agreed that with the limited funds, food prep was the best way to spend what little money we had. With the hard work they put in, the food prep staff had to have better conditions. I explained how we would be taking bids and hopefully have new cabinets in thirty days. Just as I was finishing up, a CNA came running and whispered in Regina's ear. She excused herself from the meeting and left.

Once the meeting was officially over and we were milling around, several staff asked me if I had big plans for the weekend. I looked at my watch and said, "I have dinner with my son tonight so I'll be leaving in a few minutes, right at five." The second I said those words, Regina came back and approached me.

Whispering in my ear, she said, "I thought you should know first. We just lost Lucy."

5

A month later our kitchen sparkled with new cabinets and pristine countertops. The food services staff happily skipped around as they spent the next two hours populating the new shelves with pots and pans and the various ingredients they used for cooking. Alisha was even singing while she worked. I was just returning to my office to approve the contractor's invoice when I found Melva there to greet me.

"Hey Susan, I've got some things to go over. Do have a moment?"

"Sure," I said. She'd really hit the ground running and had found numerous things we weren't billing for, along with a few items we were underbilling. With so much of my time engaged in daily crisis management, it wasn't until now that I was able to turn my attention to getting our finances in order.

Melva handed me a two-page document detailing our billings. "See the middle section? This is the final billing for the three residents we lost. We've been paid for the first two, but it doesn't look like we'll be getting anything for the last."

I looked at Lucy's name and knew I would remember her forever—she was the first resident I'd ever lost. After she died, two more had passed. "Sure, I see it. So that's all we can anticipate for reimbursement? It doesn't seem like much."

"Yes, that's it. We maxed out on them. They were all on Medicaid."

"Okay," I said, "What's this?"

"The RUG rate for the two new residents we just got in."

RUG stands for 'Resource Utilization Group.' It's something I believe we were never destined to fully understand yet it ruled our lives. RUG was a software program run by the state of Texas that required the staff to enter excruciating detail on each new resident. Once that was entered it would magically spit out the resident's RUG rate, otherwise known as the daily reimbursement from the state. This allowed the administrator to set a budget for the home. Finding out the RUG rate for each new resident was always an eventful happening since we were always hoping for a big payout. In the beginning it felt like a lottery—very random. Over time, however, we became able to fairly predict how new residents would be ranked. The lowest level was called walkie-talkies—they walked and talked, so they brought in a very low RUG rate. Those having a long list of medical issues were at the other end of the spectrum and therefore brought in a lot of money for the home.

The two new residents we'd just taken in—one of which had twelve different diagnoses of medical conditions—were big hitters. "Wow," I said. "Mr. Gendron has a 205. That's a jackpot! I guess being on a ventilator is the ticket."

"Yeah, and Mrs. Hettis snagged a 198 with all those meds and daily IVs."

I sighed. "You know, it's a strange business making money off of folks' illnesses. But that's healthcare for you. It takes some getting used to." I returned to the form. "Hey what's this? Have we actually gone down in daily reimbursements since I started?"

Melva frowned. "Unfortunately, the two we just added don't make up for the three we've lost."

I ran a hand through my hair. "Gosh, it seems one step forward and two steps back. Are we ever going to make progress?"

"We have to pay the cabinet contractor, too. Don't forget that."

"Thanks for reminding me," I said sarcastically. "Have you sent this report to Billy?"

"No, it's going out in the mail tonight."

"He'll probably go ballistic."

Melva chuckled. "You know at some point he's gonna smoke that final cigarette, hack that final cough, and drop to his knees, clutching his chest before he keels over and dies. Then we'll be dealing with someone else."

"That's scary, too. You're just brightening my day."

She smiled. "Look at line eighty-five, see that?"

"Sure, that's Mr. Hinton. He's bringing in a pretty penny. And he's only fifty-six years old."

"Right, because he's a vet. See, the VA pays top dollar for him to get a private room. It all depends on his rank, years of service and if he served in a war. You always want VA money. It's the gold standard of government reimbursements. It even beats several of the private insurance plans."

"Wow, I didn't know that. I really appreciate you educating me. With you on the staff it's like having my own mentor."

"Thanks. But speaking of Mr. Hinton, I saw the police here last week. They were in his room. Do you know what that was about?"

"Oh, nothing really. They said he was a potential witness to an incident that happened two years ago and they wanted to question him about it. I started thinking he may have been in this home when the incident happened, so I looked at his records to make sure they had the right guy and they did because he came to this home a few months after they say he witnessed it, whatever *it* is."

Melva made some notes. "I see. Well that's all I have. I better get back to it." She rose and opened the door to my office. To our surprise, the same detective who'd been questioning Mr. Hinton last week was standing right outside the door. "Oh!" Melva blurted out. "You scared me!"

"Sorry about that," the detective said. "I was just about to knock." He looked over Melva's shoulder. "Ms. Hodges, can I talk to you a moment?"

"Sure, Detective Brown. Have a seat." He waited for Melva to leave and then closed the door.

Placing his hands on my desk, he said, "First, you can call me Rhett."

I smiled, noticing he wasn't married. "Okay Rhett, what can I do for you?"

"I need to know about any health issues Mr. Hinton has."

I paused for a moment and considered his request. "I'm afraid I can't do that. HIPAA prevents us from releasing that information to anyone other than a medical provider."

"I figured you'd say that, so I brought this." Grinning, he handed me a sheaf of papers.

"What's this?"

"An arrest warrant, an affidavit of probable cause, and a request from the sheriff for his medical records. He's gonna be residing in jail for the foreseeable future."

I dropped the documents on my desk. "What?! Are you kidding me? What's the charge?"

"Murder, I'm afraid."

I closed my eyes and shook my head several times. "Murder?! So you're taking him away right now? For good?"

"For good, or at least until he can make bond. But chances are zero with his financial condition. In just a few minutes there will be two uniforms coming to take him in."

I couldn't believe what I was hearing. Mr. Hinton was a kind, gentle soul who didn't seem capable of hurting anyone. "Can you tell me what happened?"

"I'll boil it down for you. Mr. Hinton is married to a Mrs. Hinton. She claims a man raped her, but she didn't tell Mr. Hinton. Apparently she didn't want to get him upset. Instead, she told their son. The son became enraged and refused to let this man get away with it, so he set up a ruse to have the man come back over to the Hinton's house. When the man arrived, the son, his girlfriend and Mrs. Hinton surprised him. The son and the son's girlfriend then severely beat the man. Through all of this Mr. Hinton, who was apparently on medication at the time, was asleep. When they were done beating the man, they woke up Mr. Hinton and asked him what they should do with the injured man. Mr. Hinton said something to the effect of 'Well, he doesn't look worse than any beating I've ever taken. He seems fine to me. Just take him home.' So the son and his girlfriend loaded up the victim in their car and instead of taking him home, dumped him in an abandoned house. He died there. It took us a while to sort it all out, but when we did the son's girlfriend confessed. She gave up the son and Mrs. Hinton, who then gave up Mr. Hinton. So Mr. Hinton is going downtown for awhile."

I took another minute to think through all of this. "Okay, here are his medical records. I'll make a complete copy for you. Keep in mind he was a pilot in Vietnam and had a connection with Agent Orange, or at least that's what the VA doctors think. Really, he's in bad shape and I just know your jail is going to have to spend some big money keeping him healthy. If the judge allows it, we could keep him here pending the trial. We're getting reimbursed by the VA. That may save the sheriff some huge bucks."

"Thanks, that's actually a good idea and I'll pass it on. I suppose he's not likely to make a run for the border now, is he?"

"No, he stays in bed a good portion of the week. We try to get him out in a wheelchair once a day for a meal, but that's not always possible. I suggest that when you arrest him you take him out in a wheelchair—he can't really walk, or at least not far. Truthfully, I doubt he'll live out a long sentence."

The detective pulled out another copy of the warrant. "He has no criminal record, so he's eligible for probation. I have a feeling you may see him back quicker than you think. But it's up to a judge."

Right then the two officers showed up, so I excused myself to make copies while they arrested Mr. Hinton. The residents seemed to droop even further at the sight of watching one of their own wheeled out in handcuffs. For me, we were losing a top dollar resident. It seemed like this whole place was snake bitten. Each bad incident made me wonder what was next. Unfortunately, I didn't have to wait long.

The next crisis happened around 3 p.m.—shift change. No one had showed up to replace the staff going off shift, and the ones finished with their day couldn't leave because a deluge of rain was hitting the area hard. No one felt safe running for the bus in this nasty weather, so they gathered in the lobby waiting for a break. I started wondering what would happen if they left and the new staff failed to show up. Was that possible?

We all stood watching the sheets of rain when Carlos appeared, pushing several mop buckets in front of him. He dropped them off at the lobby and went back to fetch a huge load of rags that used to be towels for the residents. "What's all this?" I asked.

Carlos pointed to the street. "When it rains hard this place floods. See the way the street slopes down to the lobby and this whole side of the building? In the courtyard, the water's about to start rushing in. It's gonna be a bad one."

I went to the dining area and looked out at the lake forming in our backyard. Cigarettes butts were floating on the surface. Incredibly, it appeared whitecaps were forming. I stood transfixed as the water rushed in through the patio doors and onto the floor.

"Carlos," I yelled. "Bring those towels!"

He came running. "We're gonna need the blankets too. I'd better go get 'em."

I didn't hesitate. "Yeah, go get them!"

Several staff members came to help as we dropped to our knees and began soaking up the water as quickly as it rushed in. One of them brought over the two mop buckets, which allowed us to wring out the towels and use them again. An off duty CNA pitched in with the mop, but he quickly abandoned it once he found it couldn't pick up much water. When Carlos returned with the blankets and unfurled them, I could tell they could soak up more water than a hundred mops. Working feverishly, we soon had a makeshift dam set up near the patio doors and were just managing to keep the water at bay. With the mop buckets on the other side of the dam, we were able to soak up the escaping water. Then I heard another call for help.

I jogged to the lobby and found that the water was creeping under the front door. Several residents in the rooms along the exterior wall had their heads poking out their doors, waving for help. The water was coming in there too. It was a complete flooding.

On my knees in the lobby next to Carlos, I said, "Tell me this happens once a year, please!"

Carlos kept his head down and said, "I've been here three months and this is the second time it's happened."

"Oh man," I cried. "This is terrible!"

Carlos glanced sideways at me. "But that's not the worst of it. I need you to handle this while I climb up on the roof to push the water off. The water collects in several areas up there, and if I don't clear it the roof could collapse. It's that dangerous."

I looked up at the ceiling tiles, imagining all the water collecting above. Right at that moment two more residents yelled out, pointing to leaks in the ceiling. A food service worker was already running with trashcans to collect the dripping water.

"Go now, Carlos! Before it gives way!"

He sprung to his feet and ran to the ladder, remaining on the roof for an entire hour. Since no one could go anywhere, the trapped food service workers made dinner for both the residents and staff. At 9 p.m. the rain slacked off, allowing us to catch up and empty all the water into a street drain outside. There were a few more brief squalls, but they finally ended around 10 p.m. This allowed the staff to finally leave, though only three new workers had showed up for the next shift. I spent the next hour shuttling staff to the bus stop in my trusty Chevy, since the streets and sidewalks were too flooded to walk there. I barely made it without stalling out. It was during one of these trips that I learned the buses stopped running at midnight, something I'd never thought of. At least they resumed at 4 a.m. I guess those four hours made some kind of difference.

By midnight the residents were asleep and things were mostly back to normal. I could finally head home after dropping off a bedraggled Carlos at his apartment. I'd also left a note telling the staff

I might be a little late the next morning—or actually this morning. The ones still there laughed, wishing me good luck getting home on the flooded streets. When I finally made it home, I laid down in bed and remembered pulling the blankets up to my chin, but not much else. I was down for the count.

A week later it was time for another dinner with Vicki. She'd gotten a job with a nursing home in Arlington, close to where I lived and I wanted to hear all about it. After we ordered our meals, Vicki filled me in. "We have a 200-bed capacity with 172 residents, unless I've lost one on the drive over. It's basically a middle class home with a few upper class residents who ran through their money too fast and downsized to our home. The staff is pretty decent, but the turnover is horrendous."

"I know. My turnover rate is bad too. It seems like the staff can quit at any time and there will always be a job waiting for them somewhere else."

"Exactly. The BOM told me that for fifty cents more an hour, she's gone. It really affects the residents."

"What about your government money?"

"For reimbursements, we have about 30% Medicaid, a couple of VA residents, a few private pay and the rest are private insurance plans. The facility is in really good shape and we have a great activities director who keeps the residents occupied. I'm happy, except that each day I feel like I'm in over my head, like I don't belong there. Unlike you, I don't have the years of experience in other industries to help out."

I laughed. "Don't put too much stock in to all that experience. Each day I'm surprised I make it through to quitting time. If someone turned this into a TV series no one would believe it. I mean, the police are the main visitors for crying out loud! I'm thinking of having a separate law enforcement sign-in sheet."

It was Vicki's turn to laugh. "That flood thing sounded biblical. What happened afterwards?"

"We spent the next day mopping and wringing out the towels and blankets. Then we washed everything and put them away for the next flood. The backyard is a virtual a mud pit. The only good news is that the residents at Warm Heart can't come up to the fence and shout obscenities because their walkers get stuck in the mud. But that's the only good news. Everything else is in terrible shape."

The waitress brought our meals and we ate while Vicki went through her thoughts on each of her staff members. She then asked me about mine.

"They're mostly good people. The problem is that they're set in their ways. They've essentially institutionalized the residents and want to keep them in a specific routine that seems to paralyze them. They're like animals. The bell rings and they eat. If something causes problems for the staff, they either discourage the resident from doing it or they prevent it outright—anything that will work easier for them. I don't like it. Hopefully the new BOM can help me turn this ship around. Although God knows, it's a long turning radius. First I have to get more residents. Maybe you can afford to lose a few."

"No way," Vicki said. "I'm not letting any of mine go. They're too valuable. Unless you want the ones with low RUG rates."

"Yeah, I'll pass. We have plenty of those."

After a bit more wine I found myself getting philosophical. "You know, it's sad that we wish for residents who need a lot of care just so we can get a high RUG rate and turn a profit. It's not as if the walkie-talkies don't need help, too. One fall and they either die or turn into a high RUG rate. But no one wants them until they've crashed and need a lot of services."

"I agree. It's pretty messed up, but that's the healthcare industry for you. The doctors are going to tell a seventy-five-year-old that he should have that knee replacement because they make money doing it. 'Go ahead, sir, and have your prostate removed. Or maybe we can do that bladder surgery now.' Sure, they may live ten more years with a good quality of life, but usually it's a short time before things begin to crater. A person spends 30% of their entire healthcare dollars on the last year of life. It's amazing. Too bad we can't do anything about it."

I lifted my wine glass. "Actually, we can as soon as you can tell me when each person's last year is."

"Good point! I'll let you know when I can do that."

We clinked glasses and enjoyed the rest of the evening, putting RUG rates and holy floods out of our minds.

6

fter three full months at the Jones-Simms Nursing Center, I had enough knowledge and experience to start making some real changes. I had analyzed the shift changes and bus schedules of the seventy-five staff members and decided to start there. My first big change was to move the start of the first shift to 6 a.m., which meant it would end at 2 p.m. The second shift would now begin at 2 p.m. and run until 10 p.m. That left the final shift from 10 p.m. to 6 a.m. I thought these changes would better serve both the residents and the employees, especially during the first two shifts when most of the residents were awake. Because the third shift was so late, the staff had next to no contact with the residents. This allowed them to deal with what few problems and emergencies popped up. It also allowed me to reduce staff during the nighttime shift and load up more workers during the other two. The first shift especially needed it, as there were two meals to be prepared with the residents needing a lot of help getting up. Starting the first shift at 6 a.m. gave the nurses and food service staff time to get ready for the residents when they started waking up. After all, that's when they needed the most help.

It was no surprise that the staff resisted the shift changes. I found them very rigid and inflexible in their thinking. They looked at things from their point of view—what's easier for them. They saw Jones-Simms Nursing Center as a cold and gray institution. I looked at it as a colorful, vibrant home. Unfortunately, the staff was pushing their vision onto me much harder than I was pushing my vision onto them. I felt like a small wave rushing back out to sea, just as a large one was coming in towards the shore. This was mainly due to the fact that it was hard to find employees who wanted to work in the Red Nine area at the very low wages we paid. As a result, the ones that we could hire held more cards than I did.

Carlos and I were the only two who were on call 24/7. If an emergency happened, he had to get to work. This was a problem since he didn't own a car. Fortunately, most maintenance emergencies could wait until he arrived each morning. I, on the other hand, didn't have that luxury. I was called in during the third shift at least twice a month, with issues ranging from a stopped up toilet to problems with the residents at Warm Heart. This was a constant headache. Every few days there were confrontations. I tried contacting their LNFA, but my messages were never returned. There was a deep hatred between our facilities. Red Man and Blackie seemed to always be in the middle of it. Of course, I knew our own people were just as guilty. What I found strange, though, was that most of our staff were indifferent to the incidents, if not actively encouraging the hostilities. One person explained it like this, "They think their home is better than ours. It's like two rival high schools or something. No one is gonna let their place be dissed." I thought the whole thing was childish, but I couldn't be everywhere all the time. As a result, things happened that I had no ability to stop. Sure, I could've written up the staff and eventually fired them, but I was grateful they showed up each day (which truthfully wasn't a common occurrence). Sadly, I held a weaker hand.

One Wednesday at 10:15 p.m., I received a call while I was getting ready for bed. When I answered it, Jenny, the third shift nurse blurted out, "Oh my God, I walked into Mrs. Rose's room and Mr. Grinnell was laying on top of her going at it. They couldn't even hear that I was there and had no idea I was seeing all . . . *that!* It was completely horrible!"

"What did you do?"

"I just ran out the door and called you!"

I knew the third shift had a lot of inexperienced employees and Jenny was one of them. It was time for a teaching moment. "That was the wrong move. What you should've done is slowly backed out of their bedroom, closed their door, and stayed out of there."

"What?! I have to get some people in there to stop them!"

"No Jenny, you don't! And you won't. They are consenting adults. We are running a home, not a prison. They are residents and this is *their* home. We are guests in it. They have every right to be sexually active. Remember, you're entering their bedroom, a private and personal space. Leave them alone until you're sure they are finished. Then you can proceed with any necessary nursing care. These are situations you must train your staff to handle properly because, again, a person's desires don't die when they enter a nursing home. Understand?"

She hesitated. "Yes, I hear what you're saying, but c'mon. This just feels so wrong. You know?"

"No, I don't, Jenny. And one day you won't either. But until that day comes, we are licensed by the state of Texas. What they're doing is a right the residents have. You must follow my orders or we'll be in big trouble. If that happens you'll be on the front end of that trouble. Understand?"

"Yes, ma'am. I'll talk to the staff right now. But don't blame me if the entire home turns into a orgyfest." She mumbled something I couldn't make out just as I bid her goodnight and hung up. Training the staff was my job and, obviously, she hadn't been trained for that situation. I made a mental note to talk to my nurses the next morning about the birds and the bees and other adult privileges. Then I turned out the light on another long day of running the Jones-Simms Nursing Center.

The next morning, I was strolling around the facility—something I tried to do several times a day—and saw several of our residents out on the patio enjoying their 'after breakfast' smoke. Then I noticed three residents up against the fence shouting and pointing in the direction of Warm Heart. Racing through the door, I yelled out, "Hey, get away from the fence! Leave those people alone."

One of them looked around, apparently the only one who had heard me. He nudged the other two, who slowly twisted their heads in my direction. Immediately their smiles were replaced by guilty, downcast looks. When I got to the fence, I saw Red Man and Old Blackie on the other side with several others I'd learned to recognize. They were all shouting obscenities with cigarettes hanging from their mouths, shooting the bird just like before. I herded our three culprits away from the fence and thoroughly chastised each of them as they made their way back to the patio. Shaking my head in disgust, I went back inside. Then I heard something else. Back on the patio the residents were applauding the three heroes. That's when I realized I wasn't going to be able to stop this nonsense. In fact, I gave up and just let them go at it. Besides, no one was picking up rocks and throwing them. Hopefully, no one had a gun.

That afternoon I had a meeting with my BOM, Melva. One of our residents, Ms. Huey, was reaching the end of her . . . *money*. This was always a difficult situation in the nursing home business. First, Ms. Huey had been admitted to our facility under Medicare. Medicare paid 100% of everything—including a private room—so she had had nothing to worry about. After twenty days were up, however, Medicare dropped to covering only 80% of the costs. Fortunately, she had a supplemental policy with Blue Cross/Blue Shield, which picked up the remaining 20%. With private insurance, Ms. Huey had nothing to worry about . . . for seventy-nine more days.

Medicare will pay some amount for nursing home care up to one hundred days. After that, the party's over. And not just for Ms. Huey, but for us as well. That's when we have to do the move—wheeling her bed from a private room into that of another resident's. For folks with no supplemental insurance, they go semi-private after the first one hundred days.

But here's where it gets even tougher: at some point, and it might be one hundred days, insurance companies like Blue Cross/Blue Shield will drop to 5%. That's what happened to Ms. Huey. She had to start draining her assets, which had started at $25,000. It didn't take long to fall to the dreaded $2,000 cutoff. When that happens, Medicaid will kick-in and pay for the remainder of the costs—up to 100% if necessary. But Medicaid is brutal. They have armies of folks who spend serious time looking for any assets they can seize. *Anything!* If the resident receives social security, which most do, they direct the entire social security check to go to the nursing home to help pay for her care, except $30 to $60. Then Medicaid will pay the nursing home the balance of her bill after social security is applied. They're like a governmental vacuum cleaner, sucking up anything they can find. I suppose as a loyal taxpayer, I should be glad they're working hard and saving me money, making sure no one is getting a free ride when they can actually afford to pay. But on the flipside people like me see the harsh realities, the merciless face of nursing home poverty. Right now, that's where Ms. Huey was. She had run out of both Medicare and private insurance and had drained her money dry. Now, she was done. It was Medicaid for the rest of her life, along with strict financial controls. The second her account crept over $2,000, they denied her Medicaid. Thus Medicaid doesn't allow a resident to simply get their social security check, cash it and blow the money on clothes or family. No, it's truly like prison where the resident can only spend so much money a month. Need to buy some more deodorant? Sorry. Wait two months. Need some new shirts? Wait four months. That's how strict it is.

Our job was to make sure Ms. Huey didn't break any Medicaid rules and get kicked out of the program. If that happened, we'd lose the money they were paying us and Mrs. Huey, too. One less resident meant a greater loss to our mother ship. It was tough. But when they pay, you play by their rules.

I was looking through her financial sheet when I saw something that puzzled me. "Hey, what's this?"

Melva looked at where I was pointing. "Oh that's the $45 for the court. They suck that out of her account first, even before Medicaid if you can believe that."

"So what's the $45 for?"

"Court."

I stared at Melva, trying to see if she was being funny. "Court? That's doesn't tell me anything. Did she have some kind of judgment she has to pay off?"

Melva shifted in her chair. "Uh, well, I really don't know. It started a few years after I began my last job. At first it was one resident, then it was a couple. By the time I left it was a whole bunch. It's the local probate court. They're removing $45 from residents' accounts and where it goes, I have no idea. I've asked before and no one ever gave me an answer that made sense."

I looked at the $45 again. "That's odd. I mean, it's not a lot of money, but it's $540 a year times however many residents. Is Ms. Huey the only one who has to pay it?"

Melva studied her list. "No, we have seven residents who pay it."

"Wow! That's almost $4,000 a year. We could sure use that money for improvements, or at least the residents could. I'll do some checking and see what I can find out."

I ended my day a few hours later and headed home. At 8 p.m. my phone rang. Thirty seconds later I slammed the phone down and five minutes later I was in my car headed back to the facility. This sounded bad. Real bad.

I rushed into the home and I saw my head nurse waiting for me. "Come into my office and fill me in."

As soon as the door closed, she started. "Okay, it's like this. One of our CNAs, Beth, walked into Ms. Huey's room, the one she used to share with Mrs. Naranjo. (Mrs. Naranjo had recently died.) That's when she saw Wayne (another CNA) in there on top of Mrs. Huey. When he heard Beth come into the room, he rolled off the bed and tried to get up, but his pants were pulled down to his ankles. They caught on Mrs. Huey's foot and he fell to the floor. Beth went around the bed and saw him lying there, butt-naked. I mean, she saw *everything!*"

I blinked a few times as I processed what she was saying. Fortunately I was able to formulate a question. "What was Mrs. Huey doing?"

"Beth said she was just lying there, kinda in shock or just takin' it. It's hard to say. She's pretty quiet, anyway."

"Where is Wayne right now?"

"I just checked and he's back doing his rounds like nothin' happened."

"Does he know you called me?"

"Yeah, I think so."

"Okay, go get Beth. But do it calmly and slowly like no big deal. Make sure you aren't around Wayne when you tell her. Got it?"

"Yes, ma'am. I got it."

Once she was gone I put my head in my hands trying to comprehend this. After a few moments, I grabbed Wayne's employment file and scanned through it. Then my head nurse showed up with the witness. Beth confirmed almost word for word what I'd just heard from her boss. I told my head nurse that when Wayne was in my office, I wanted both of them and another registered nurse to stay by Mrs. Huey until I came for them. I didn't want anything else to happen. With that in place, I got up and went to look for Wayne.

I found him working hard, folding towels near the laundry room. "Wayne, how are you doing?"

He grinned at me with an innocent look. "Great, Ms. Hodges. How are you?" The staff rarely called me Ms. Hodges, so this was a signal that he knew there was a problem.

"I'm good." That was a lie. Actually, I was freaking out. "Can I please talk to you in my office?"

"Sure, no problem," he said with another false grin.

Once we reached my office I told him to have a seat and then closed the door.

I opened his file. "I understand we had an incident and I may have to document your file on this, so I want to be clear on exactly what happened."

He licked his dry lips. "Well, I was tending to Mrs. Huey when Beth walked in. That was about it."

I made some notes. "Okay. Did you have your pants down?"

Wayne hesitated, his eyes narrowing on a speck of dust located on the floor.

"Look," I said, "don't lie to me. Your record shows you've been selected as the CNA of the year three times and you've been here practically the longest of anyone. I don't like losing good people so tell me the truth and I'll decide your punishment . . . *if any.*"

The hope of scraping through all of this unscathed seemed to jar him loose. "Okay, here's what's going on. Mrs. Huey and I are in love. She consented to have sex and I really love her."

I made some notes while appearing calm. "I see. But she's sixty-eight and you're thirty-four. Does that make sense? Really?"

He leaned towards me. "I know it's hard for you to understand, but we have a special connection. I love her."

"But does she love you?"

"Yes, she does!"

I kept making notes. "All right, I want you to take this piece of paper and write up everything and let me look at it. Then I'll decide what to do. Understand?"

"Yes, ma'am."

He took the paper and started writing. When he was done he handed it back to me. Sure enough, he had admitted to having sex, claimed it was consensual and that they loved each other. Just reading it made me want to throw up. At the same time I knew showing any reaction could be dangerous. There was no telling what someone like him might do if he thought he was going to be punished. And I was most definitely going to punish him. Very shortly.

"This looks fine, Wayne. Now, go back to work and stay away from Mrs. Huey or any of the other female residents until I decide what I'm going to do. Understand?"

He nodded. "I understand, Ms. Hodges. But are you gonna tell my wife? She'd have a big problem with all this."

"I don't think I have that right. You're an employee and I don't think I can discuss employment issues with her. So don't worry, I won't be talking to her. If she finds out, it surely won't be from me." I forced a smile.

He exhaled loudly. "Oh thank God! That would've been bad."

I continued smiling and nodding. "Yes, I'm sure it would've been. Now go back to work. You're off shift in one hour, right?"

"Yes, one hour."

"Okay. I'll have a decision before then so you won't have to stress about it all night." I let him out the door and watched him confidently stroll back to the laundry room. Then I kept up my casual veneer as I walked back to my office and calmly closed the door. As soon as I heard the lock catch, I couldn't get to the phone fast enough.

"9-1-1, what's your emergency?"

Five minutes later, two officers came bursting into the lobby where I stood waiting. I briefly told them about what had happened and they demanded to find Wayne immediately. Within moments he was safely detained while a third officer arrived and talked to me in my office. After he read Wayne's statement, he went to talk to Mrs. Huey. A few minutes later I watched a handcuffed Wayne led out of the facility. That relieved confident look he had when he left my office was long gone. I could tell he was no longer worried about what his wife would think and was considering how all this would look to twelve strangers.

Once he was gone, the police called an ambulance to take Mrs. Huey to the hospital, where they proceeded to perform a rape kit examination on her. I went home and got a wink of sleep before the sun peeped through my curtains, alerting me that it was time to get up and deal with the enormous weight of this situation. I came in with deep bags under my eyes and was just situated at my desk when Billy called me. After I explained everything to him, he began coughing. "Crap! Things like this are bad, not to mention terrifying for Mrs. Huey. I understand you took her to the hospital?"

"Yes, they examined her and admitted her for the night. We're picking her up this morning and she'll be back here in thirty minutes."

"Oh boy. This means a potential lawsuit from her family, not to mention DADS crawling up our ass. We have to notify the state today. I'll have the staff do that from here." He held the phone away while he coughed hard.

"What do you want me to do? I assume we need to terminate Wayne?"

When he regained his voice, he said, "Yeah, we'll do that from here too. You fax in everything and the girls will handle it. God this is bad. I guess it's time for Sid."

"Who's Sid?"

"See that piece of neon pink paper on the wall next to the list of phone numbers?"

I stared at a well-worn list of corporate phone numbers that had been there long before I started. Sure enough, next to it was a neon pink post-it, something I'd never noticed before. "Sure, I see it. There's just a phone number on it."

"That's right, but it's a very important number. When you hang up with me, call it and ask for Sid. Tell him I told you to call. Then tell him everything. Okay?"

"Sure, but what's this all about?"

"Look Susan, just do it. Okay? He'll start airdrops of water on this forest fire while I pull out the pins of some Texas-sized fire extinguishers and spray foam on this ass whipping that's coming. Goodbye!" *Click.*

Shaking my head in confusion, I dialed the number and a rough voice answered. "Yeah?"

It wasn't the professional sounding voice I expected. "Is Sid there?"

"Do you work for Billy?"

This was odd. "Uh, yes."

"Figures. That son-of-a-bitch can never get it right. It sounds like sip, like sipping a vodka tonic. Get it?"

"Oh sorry. *Sip* then. Billy said to call you."

He started coughing, which made me wonder if he wasn't Billy's brother. "Okay. It must be a big problem, right?"

"Yes, it is."

"Fine. Tell me the problem in one sentence."

I paused a moment to collect my erratic thoughts. "Sure, well . . . let's see . . . one sentence. Okay. My three-time CNA of the year just raped a sixty-eight-year-old resident."

"Fine," he said, without surprise or shock. "You got a pen? Write this down." I fumbled for a pen as he started spitting out a street name. Just as I finished writing down the last digit of the address, he said, "I'll see you in one hour."

"Wait! How much do you charge?"

"More than you can afford." *Click.*

I sat there bewildered. It was all very strange, like something out of a movie. But unlike a movie, we were on a tight budget. I didn't want to get underwater with some high-priced consultant. Still, Billy did say to contact him. And I had been an LNFA for less than six months, which meant I didn't have much experience in dealing with something like this. So I just had to go with it, though nothing could've prepared me for where that meeting would lead me. Nothing!

7

I made it to the Meadowbrook area of Fort Worth and drove down streets lined with large, mature trees. Many of the current homes were built in the 1970s. At one time this was a suburb where young professionals with money had come to build large homes on even larger lots and play golf at the local course. But even though there were pockets of homes being updated, like most neighborhoods over time the area had transitioned downward. I glanced down at the address on my piece of paper and slowed in front of a one-story, painted brick house. That's when my inner voice clicked in. I'd talked to the man for less than two minutes and now I was meeting him at his house to discuss the rape of our sixty-eight-year-old resident. As a woman, I should've been more concerned, but for some reason I wasn't. I trusted Billy and assumed this man would help me with any problems we had to face.

Grabbing my small bag of notes and documents, I locked the car and strode up the sidewalk to the door with a sense of urgency that transferred into my knocks. Hearing nothing in return, I was just raising my fist to knock again when the door opened.

"Are you Susan?"

Standing before me was a tall man, probably 6'-6", slightly over-weight, with a trimmed gray beard to match his trimmed gray hair. He wore jeans and a shirt that looked like they were on their second day, although it could've been because he'd been up all night. It was hard to tell. "Yes," I said presenting my hand. "I'm Susan Hodges."

He shook it and grumbled. "C'mon in and let's get after it."

I followed him into the living room where he had a large desk and table piled high with various folders and papers. The place looked like an office, except it was his home. A TV on mute sat opposite his desk. After taking a seat, I waited for him to get organized.

Glancing around, the place looked like a maid came through and cleaned once a week. It smelled faintly like cigarettes, but certainly not as bad as what I assumed Billy's home must smell like. I handed him some documents with a yellow post-it displaying his name in big letters. He ripped off the post-it and held it up. "It's spelled S-Y-P, not S-I-P."

"Oh sorry, I didn't know."

"Why should you? Especially when Billy calls me Sid."

I made a quick note, although I don't know if it mattered all that much in comparison to what we were dealing with. "Okay, *Syp*, I got it. Is that short for something?" I wanted to take the words back as soon as they left my mouth. This man didn't appear to be the kind who got into small talk, yet here I was trying to engage him when I should've just shut up and let him take over.

"No, it's not short for anything. It stands for Solve Your Problem. S-Y-P."

"Okay," I said, deciding against any extra commentary.

He cleared his throat. "Now, let's get down to your Wayne here. DADS will be out tomorrow. That means you have the rest of to-day to get ready. Here's a list of things they'll be looking for. If you need to keep staff late and pay overtime, do it. Make sure you check each item thoroughly and are in complete compliance. Understand?"

"Yes," I said looking over the items. "I understand."

"Now, the person coming out will be female. She'll have an at-titude, but when she finds the first five items in compliance, she'll lighten up. Do you have any fresh flowers set out?"

"No, but I can get some."

"Don't. She's allergic to flowers and pollen in general. Do not have fresh flowers anywhere, understand?"

"No problem. I'll make sure we don't have any." With the financial situation we had, there was no money for flowers anyway, nor ice sculptures for that matter.

He flipped through the pages of the folder I'd just handed him. "Does this file contain the relatives of Mrs. Huey?"

"Yes, it does."

He continued looking. "Good. It has their visits listed here, which appear to be a few times a year. I can take care of that." I wasn't sure what he meant about 'taking care of that.' Dropping the folder, he said, "Any questions?"

Now it was my turn to clear my throat. "Well, sure. What's going to happen? Who's coming out?"

"If you follow my instructions to the letter, DADS will be the only agency coming out. Once they issue a report, we'll see what it says. Hopefully they'll go light on you. Of course, the police will come back to get more statements. They may also call you and some of your staff down to the station. You must cooperate fully, especially since there may have been another staff member who was an accomplice. You know, a lookout. That kind of thing."

I swallowed hard. "Gosh, I hadn't thought about that."

"Yeah, you haven't thought about a lot of things because you don't have enough experience yet."

I nodded, even though he was being somewhat rude. "You're right about that. I assume you know the ins and outs of this industry, huh?"

"Yes, I do. I know every nook and cranny in the nursing home business, but only in Texas. Other states? No way. But Texas I got nailed. That's why folks like Billy get me involved when there's a problem. I'm sure you and I will be dealing with each other many more times, especially with your facility located in the Red Nine area."

That wasn't a pleasant thought. "I was hoping this would be the first and last one. Then again, I've already dealt with several shocking events, so you may be right."

"Yeah, like Mr. Hinton arrested for murder?"

"Oh, you know about that?"

"I sure do. That's how I get paid—to know things. I float around in the background while you get all the hard work done. Any more questions?"

I thought about keeping my mouth shut, but simply couldn't. "Actually yes. There's a $45 charge being taken from Mrs. Huey's account. What's that for?"

He glanced at the page. "That's the probate court. They control her assets by court order and take the $45 to run their program."

"Oh, okay. I just wanted to make sure it was legitimate." I started getting my things together, but he had more to say.

"I didn't say it's legit. It's *legal,* but far from legit."

I stopped and stared at him. "I don't understand."

"Of course you don't understand. You're in my generation. Do you remember seeing a movie from the late seventies called *Coma?*

"I think so. Maybe."

"Well, you brush up on that movie and when you do, during the next crisis we'll talk more about your $45 concern. Now, you've got a lot to do, so you'd better get on with it."

"Yes, sir. Thanks again."

He said nothing as he closed the door behind me.

That was interesting, I thought to myself. This job certainly was full of strange experiences.

Ten days later I received the DADS report detailing the results of their survey. It had no violations and the whole thing had gone down just like Syp had predicted. Then and there I gained tremendous respect for him. The guy obviously knew his stuff and by following his instructions, the truth was laid bare for everyone to see, including the inspectors. No one could argue with the truth, not even DADS. Strange as he was, Syp was the kind of guy I wanted on my team—one who wasn't afraid of laying out the whole truth.

With this report finished, our statements to the police and the termination of Wayne, the matter was effectively concluded. I was relieved. The entire ordeal was tough for the staff and most of all, for Mrs. Huey. She needed a lot of help. The only good news out of all this was that ten months later Wayne was convicted of Aggravated Sexual Assault and sentenced to eight years in prison. He wouldn't be raping any more women in nursing homes again. Plus, they had his DNA in a registry for any future rapes. Good riddance!

I made it somehow to New Year's Eve. We were about to turn the page on this tumultuous year, but before I could spend time hoping for a better one next year I still had a lot of work to do. Unfortunately, this last day had a very unpleasant task.

Melva greeted me with the paperwork I didn't want to see. "Oh no, do we have to go through with this today?"

She sat down and said, "I'm okay with letting it slide if you are. Remember, you run things here, not me. And today I'm damn glad."

"To tell you the truth, I've been dreading this moment. Really dreading it. This has got to be one of the toughest things I've ever done."

"I hear you. I did it many times when I was an admin. It never gets easy."

The problem I didn't want to face had a name, and it was Mrs. Costello. She was a human being who deserved respect. She had feelings—feelings I was about to crush. However, it had to be done for the good of our facility and the company. After all, we weren't a charity. This was a for-profit enterprise, one that required money. The problem with Mrs. Costello was that she had none.

It all started just over thirty days ago. She'd been living in a house with family members and needed so much care that they couldn't keep her. They decided to put her in a nursing home and therefore called us. This is where things started going off track.

When you're poor and have absolutely no money you have to find a home that will take you. However, when we take you in we have a plan. That plan is called Medicaid. But Medicaid isn't stupid. They know folks want to game the system and get free services when they can actually pay for them. So they require you to actually be admitted to a nursing home for thirty days first, before funding you. This accomplishes several things. First, Medicaid finds out if you really want and need nursing care. During that thirty-day period the resident will sometimes leave voluntarily because they don't like living in a nursing home. Other times the nurses will discover something that will allow the resident to go back home and live independently. When that happens, Medicaid doesn't have to pay.

The second reason for the thirty-day trial period is to put the onus on the healthcare facility (us) to screen these people and make sure they have no assets. They accomplish this by not paying for these first thirty-days until the resident has become officially approved. If they don't get approved, the facility eats all of that free care. It's expensive, especially since they usually need a lot of services. And Mrs. Costello needed a lot of services. That's what made me agree to take her on. Her RUG rate was very high. All we had to do was get her approved on Medicaid.

We filled out the forms promptly and gave them to the next of kin who had to verify the information because Mrs. Costello had dementia. They took the forms home to study them and this is where we ran into a roadblock. They refused to sign and get them back to us. Plain and simple.

Now why would people fail to do that? Prison! The forms detail all of the financial transactions for the last two years and require disclosure of any money transferred during that time period. If Mrs. Costello had $100,000 and signed it over to a daughter two weeks earlier, Medicaid would go after that money as soon as they approved Mrs. Costello. The same goes for a home or other real estate. Even funeral plots are seized. Really, it's unbelievable.

Usually when we get no answer from the family (or one that doesn't make sense), rest assured we know they have the money to pay for care, but don't want to. In Mrs. Costello's case I believed she still owned the home her family was living in. That home would've been seized and the occupants evicted if they had signed the papers. That's where Melva and I came in. It was Melva's job as BOM to get each resident qualified and start the money flowing in. When she couldn't, she let me know and I had to take action. We were required by law to give a resident a thirty-day notice before we evicted them. To protect ourselves, we give each new, unqualified resident a thirty-day eviction notice the very first day they arrive, so we aren't on the hook for another thirty days. When Mrs. Costello's thirty days were up, I spent two more days calling her family and receiving assurances that they were either going to bring in her forms or coming to pick her up. Neither one happened. Some nursing homes let this go on forever until the home goes broke. I wasn't about to do that. I told the family very clearly that if she weren't picked up by December 30, she would be taken away. When December 30 came and went, we still had Mrs. Costello and they still had not given us the completed forms. They had called my bluff.

Now I had to do what I had to do. This was going to be my first 'eviction,' but sadly, not my last. The nurses placed her meds in a clear baggie and loaded her into our van. I drove her myself, partially because our driver wasn't available, but mostly to save money. The state of Texas says we have to drop the resident off at a safe place. Believe it or not, a homeless shelter falls into that category. So that's where I took her.

As I pulled up to the shelter, I had one of our nurses help Mrs. Costello out of the van and inside. When the nurse came back to the van she was cursing under breath, clearly upset about this whole process and me. In fact, the entire staff felt the same way. Many of them called me names behind my back and gave me evil looks. After all, taking a sick, old lady to a homeless shelter was a horrendous thing to do. I felt extremely bad too, but I had no choice. The alternative was to have our facility shut down and dump all the residents onto the street. Then the employees would lose their jobs. How many curses would they spit at me then?

By taking her to the homeless shelter we hoped to scare/shame the family into taking her back, but they didn't. I'd seen this happen with a dog. If a neighbor was moving into an apartment because they could no longer afford their house, they'd leave the dog in the backyard. They knew someone would eventually call animal control, who would then take the dog to an animal shelter. The shelter staff would find the owners at their new apartment and try to get them to pick up the dog. Since the apartment wouldn't accept animals, they couldn't take the dog back. Thus, the dog was eventually put down. There were a lot of parallels between our situation and that one, and it was all terribly sad. In the end, we had to leave Mrs. Costello at the shelter.

Most shelters require every person to pack up each morning and leave, then come back at a designated time and stand in line hoping to get a room for the night. If they don't get one, they sleep outside. If they're weak like Mrs. Costello, they eventually collapse. If they don't die, an ambulance comes to pick them up and take them to the hospital. There they'll be stabilized, pumped up with meds, and dumped again until they finally die from the stress. Usually though, they die the first time. But at least the family doesn't have to give up her house and assets to Medicaid. A lot of families think, "Hey, she's gonna die anyway. Why shouldn't we get her stuff?" Believe me, you see a lot of bad things in this business, but for better or worse, we never found out what happened to Mrs. Costello.

The new year started and sure enough, we were right back in the same boat with another resident. This time it was a little different. Mr. Donovan had been living at a home he owned and had some assets. His family lived with him, but had somehow caught the attention of the local probate court. The court declared Mr. Donovan incompetent, assigned a lawyer to handle his affairs and began sucking up his assets under court authority. When all this happened, up popped another $45 fee to be removed each month from his account. I still wasn't sure how all this worked and assumed it was all on the up and up. After all, it was the court system with judges, lawyers and administrative personnel. They weren't going to do anything wrong. Right? Besides, I had a lot on my plate.

I'd recently discovered a serious problem involving our controlled substances, which were kept under lock and key in a drug storage area. Like everything else at Jones-Simms, the drug storage locker needed replacing with professional cabinets and locks. It was high on my priority list and something we were going to do as soon as I got the money. The locks we had now could definitely be manipulated if one wanted to take the time and work on it. Of course, that assumed they had the time and that no one would come by and see them at it.

My director of nursing, Regina Johnson, was in charge of the controlled substance inventory. As such, she had access to all of the drugs, including one in particular—Vicodin. Vicodin is a brand name for hydrocodone. For many people, hydrocodone is highly addictive, and like most addictive drugs, can quickly ruin their lives. I first started noticing the problem when I was making my normal rounds and talking to the residents. Several complained that they were still in pain, despite receiving their usual hydrocodone pills. I made note of it and went to look at their files. After studying the matter, I talked to Regina. Her explanation was that they were building up a tolerance to the drug. She suggested waiting a few days and then we could talk to the doctor about increasing their dosage. This seemed like a good idea, especially since I knew a body could get used to a drug.

Within days though, the residents who had been complaining stopped. They seemed quite content. When I talked to each one, they assumed I'd waved my magic wand and made it all better. Yet I'd done nothing, so I was somewhat baffled as to why they were all feeling better. Then three different residents began complaining about their pain. This was odd. I pondered the matter and looked at my watch. It was near the 2 p.m. shift change, so I decided to wait until the new shift came on and everyone was knee-deep in getting the residents to dinner. That's when I quietly made my way to the drug storage locker and did an inventory of the pain pills.

The inventory sheet I printed out from my office said there were five unopened bottles of Vicodin and fifty pills gone from a 250-pill bottle. When I lifted the opened bottle, it felt heavy, like there were at least 200 pills. That was a good sign. I unscrewed the lid and looked in. Sure enough there were plenty of long white ovals with Vicodin clearly printed on each one. I poured some out and got a big surprise. Along with the Vicodin were other white oval pills lacking the Vicodin stamp. I had no idea what they were. I could tell someone had made a top layer of Vicodin to fool anyone looking into the bottle. That's when I knew I had a problem. I was about to leave the storage room, when I decided to check the unopened bottles for good measure.

Taking one down, I noticed the plastic seal was gone, but the secondary seal underneath the cap was still in place. After a careful inspection, I could see someone had glued the secondary seals back in place. To no surprise, they were full of the same blanks I'd found in the opened bottle. My heart raced as I found all five bottles of Vicodin were mostly used up. Except for the few pills covering the opened bottle, we were out of painkillers. Now I understood why the residents were in pain. Someone was taking their pills and feeding them blanks.

Since Regina had been working different shifts to make sure she was the one to dispense the pain pills, she was my primary suspect. Still, it could be someone else. Whoever was doing it, I had to catch them in the act. I put everything back just the way I'd found it and went to my office to think about how to catch the culprit. As I was brainstorming, my eyes wandered aimlessly around my office until they landed on a familiar neon-pink post-it note. That's when I knew it was time to make another call to Syp.

8

Once again I was sitting before this eccentric, somewhat out-of-place man. It looked like he was wearing the exact same clothes from my first visit. Maybe he hadn't even left his house. I had just finished telling him about the pill problem and was waiting for his response.

"Okay," he said rolling a toothpick back and forth with his tongue. "We'll start at the top and work our way down the list of suspects. It may be your director of nursing or it may be someone totally unrelated. With the shoddy storage locker you folks have, there's no telling who's been getting in there. To keep our options open, here's what I want you to do."

I pulled out my pad and wrote everything down. The plan wasn't perfect, but it just might work. Once he'd finished quizzing me over a few of the details, I decided to bring up something that had been bothering me. "I watched that movie *Coma* with Michael Douglas. It was a good movie, but I don't see how it applies to a nursing home facility or the $45 that's being taken from many of the residents' accounts."

He tossed the toothpick towards a small wastebasket and missed. "What do you think the movie was about? Boil it down into one or two sentences."

"This bad guy, who's the head of surgery for a hospital, sets up a special gas line that runs carbon dioxide into an operating room. He can turn this line on at any time and make the person brain dead. He then takes the living body to a special place where the organs are sold to the highest bidder. Sort of like a black market for organs."

Syp smiled. "Good. Very good. Except the bad guy piped in carbon *monoxide*, not carbon *dioxide*. There's a big difference."

"Sorry. But I still don't see how this applies to a $45 charge on many of our residents' accounts."

"Oh, but it does! It most certainly does. Instead of harvesting organs, the bad guys are harvesting assets. Plain and simple."

"Assets?! That's crazy. How?"

"Simple. In the movie, the patient goes in for routine surgery and ends up losing their organs. In our version, an elderly person forgets a few things and soon, their loving family goes to court to have a guardian appointed for them. The guardian immediately takes control of all of their assets, sends them to his or her buddies to manage, uses the resident's assets to pay for all that management, and before long the person is poor. Then they ship 'em out of their house or nice nursing home to some rundown facility like yours where they'll be on Medicaid until they die."

"But what about the poor people? Why does it happen to them?"

"You'd be surprised what they can do with a poor person. First, they're gonna scrape $45 from each Medicaid check. Then they'll scour anything they've ever owned or might've owned. Maybe burial plots or a piece of a home owned by a distant relative. Maybe even a potential lawsuit against a business. Anything. Then they put a law firm on them to spend, sell, or drain the assets before they go to Medicaid, because they know the Medicaid trolls will gobble it all up. It's like two hogs running towards a trough. The first one to get there eats all the food."

"That's crazy. No one's getting rich over $45!"

"What you don't understand is that they deal in volume. Like *Coma*, every organ is worth something. And I didn't tell you the best part: Texas law allows a judge to declare you incompetent without anyone filing anything. Let's say you're seventy-five years old and have a lawsuit going on in a court, but you refuse to settle. Someone whispers in the judge's ear that you're incompetent and boom! He holds a hearing, orders you to be examined by a doctor (which of course the judge selects) and bingo! You're ruled incompetent. In seconds a law firm is handling your affairs, paying themselves from your assets and performing a financial rape of your life's work. It doesn't matter if you have other doctors say you're competent. As long as one court-appointed doctor can say you're incompetent—just enough to give the judge something to hang his hat on, the same judge who's just itching to let his buddies feed at your trough—you're toast. Time to harvest your assets."

"So whether or not you're competent, the judge simply finds you incompetent so he can oversee the taking of your assets? It all sounds too far-fetched."

"Far-fetched? Ever hear of a Venus flytrap? Who'd ever think something like that exists? As soon as a fly trips the sensors, the plant closes and sucks you dry of everything—money, property and life. And at $45 bucks x 500 people x one year, that's $270,000! For a judge who makes $130,000 a year, that's a nice bonus. He'll maybe spend it on himself or perhaps hire his daughter to come in and do some filing for a nicely inflated salary. Maybe even take a trip to Fiji to attend a judicial conference. People can always find creative *and* legal ways to spend money."

"But what about the lawyers appointed to watch over these people?"

Syp put another toothpick in his mouth. "What about 'em?"

"Aren't they entrusted with an ethical duty to protect their clients?"

"Sure, and they can do the right thing. But how do you think they got their jobs in the first place?"

"I don't know. Do they apply for it? Maybe an agency has a rotating list or something."

"Wrong! The judge appoints them. They can be his close buddies or friends of his buddies. Or really anyone he wants. And guess what? The judge is an elected official. He needs to stay in office. His buddies understand this situation, so they willingly donate the money he needs to run for reelection. This means they'll get more guardianships and more assets to suck dry. They can also put the money in a bank the lawyer or judge are friends with, or better yet, a bank that supports the judge's reelection campaign. Of course, the lawyer gets paid a fee from the assets—he sends the bill to the judge who appointed him. It's no different than having a stockbroker manage your money, one who churns trades to earn tons of commissions for himself. Eventually, you run out of money. Same deal here."

"Wow! That's really hard to believe."

"Trust me, it's true. Anytime they want, they just rip the poor person from their nice, comfortable nursing home to some pigpen that's convenient. 'Oh, Mrs. Johnson is happy at ABC Nursing Home? That's too far for me to drive and see her, so in her best interests I'm having her transferred to XYZ Home right down the block from where I live. That way I can bill a weekly visit and drain her assets faster.' Who cares that Mrs. Johnson will experience trauma in moving to a new home. It's all what the lawyer wants and what makes money for the first hog at the trough."

I slapped the table. "If what you're saying is true, why doesn't someone do something about it?"

"Remember the ending of *Coma*?"

"Yeah, so?"

"Remember how the female doctor discovered this whole illegal scheme and confided in the head surgeon, except he was actually the bad guy? What did he do? He doped her up and told the staff she needed an emergency appendectomy. Then he ordered her to be taken to operating room number eight, the one with the carbon monoxide. All it takes is a 'doctor-friend' of the judge saying you're incompetent and poof! You'll be doped up and whisked away to a nursing home while your assets are devoured. Then, when you're broke, you'll end up in the Jones-Simms Nursing Center with some-one shoving a pill down your gullet three times a day to keep you brain dead. Sound familiar?"

I was sure he was exaggerating or trying to scare me for some un-known reason. Or maybe he was a bit 'touched,' as my grandmother used to say. Either way, his first plan in handling the state investiga-tion had worked great, so I had to believe him. I glanced at my watch to give him a hint that it was time for me to leave. Then to hammer home the point, I said, "Well, that's quite a story. But speaking of pills, I think I have your game plan down and I'll need to be execut-ing it shortly. I'll call and keep you updated with any developments."

He could see I was done with his conspiracy theory and remained silent while I gathered up my things. Then, just as I was about to leave, he grabbed my hand. "Susan, don't go poking around in things that don't concern you, understand? Just accept what I'm telling you and leave it alone. Don't get near operating room number eight. You hear?"

I nodded my head. "I hear you. Stay away from operating room number eight. Got it. And don't worry, I've got plenty on my plate to keep me from poking around in all that mess."

As I walked out to my car, I reminded myself to conduct more of our business on the phone. Or at least bring along another person. He might not be all there.

The first thing Syp had told me to do was to change the locks on the drug storage locker. There were only three nurses who had access to it besides me. Because the controlled drugs were stored in a sec-ond locked cabinet inside the drug storage locker, I changed that as well. Then I told each nurse that I'd be periodically changing the locks and issuing new keys to make sure copies weren't made. I pretended it was corporate policy and didn't make a big deal about it. With this move I was hoping to narrow down the list of suspects to just three. If the pill theft stopped, then chances were good it was someone else.

The next part of the plan was the keys themselves. Regina, the director of nursing, was given a real key to the second cabinet within the drug storage locker while the other two nurses were given fakes. They rarely dispensed controlled substances and wouldn't need to use them for several days, if not weeks. If they did need something before then, they'd find their key didn't work and come to me. This would give me a chance to question them. In the meantime, only Regina would have access to the second cabinet.

To flush out the addict, I told each of them we were getting in two large bottles of Vicodin, but not to open them until the others were used up since we had plenty on hand. Each bottle was sealed with plastic—it would be impossible to open them without me noticing. Following Syp's plan, each new bottle came with a nice surprise inside. I did all this late Tuesday afternoon, telling them the shipment would be in the next morning, and again, not making a big deal about it.

I got to work early the next morning and planted the bottles. Then I had Melva, who knew about the problem, follow Regina around as she dispensed the pills. Melva also knew what Vicodin looked like and was going to steal a few of the pills from the residents. (We would come back later and give the resident their medication.) Regina wasn't worried about Melva because our company had a succession plan in place and I'd made the announcement some time back that Melva would run the home when I was absent, on vacation, or got hit by a bus. Thus, each department head knew that Melva would be spending time with them to learn more about their job and the business. This gave Melva the cover she needed. With everything in place, the plan started.

To make her normal rounds, Regina first went into drug storage locker to fill up the pill cups. This took about ten minutes. When she was done, she began delivering them to the residents. Melva went with her. When Regina handed her the pill cups to dispense, Melva took the opportunity to steal a few of the Vicodin. After the rounds, Melva came to my office and showed me the pills. Sure enough they were fakes. But this didn't mean Regina was the culprit. She could've been dispensing the fake pills someone else had planted. It was possible she didn't look at them closely. That's where the final part of Syp's plan came in.

One of the other nurses who had a fake key happened to be in too. Even though she didn't have access to the controlled substance cabinet, she could get into the drug storage locker, so I had to be sure. I reached over and turned up the volume on the baby monitor I had planted in the drug storage locker. Melva joined me when her rounds were over.

"Do you think this will work?" she asked.

"It might. These things pick up any sound. If she's gonna get into it, now's her best opportunity. Especially since the pills have already been dispensed and the other nurses are occupied getting the residents to and from breakfast. If it's the other nurse, she would have to pick the lock somehow or have a duplicate key made, which would be tough since I just handed them out yesterday."

We waited ten minutes and were about to move on to some other chores when we heard a noise on the monitor. Someone had just opened up the door to the storage locker. The next noise we heard was someone jiggling the new lock. I couldn't tell if they had a key or were picking it, but I was sure they were undoing it somehow. The next sound was unmistakable: the plastic seal was being removed. We were about to catch our culprit.

I could hear the large cap being unscrewed and then a loud *boing!* This was followed by an even louder shriek. Melva and I raced out of my office to the storage locker. When Melva pulled back the door, there standing in front of me was the pill thief trying desperately to stuff the colorful spring back into the pill bottle. When she heard us, she jumped backwards in shock.

"What are you doing with those pills?" I asked.

Calmly she said, "Oh, someone played a joke on me and stuffed this spring into the bottle to scare me. Really, it's nothing. Just someone's idea of a stupid joke."

I reached over for the bottle. "Come with me to my office, Regina. We need to talk."

"But we need to lock up first."

"Don't worry, Melva will do that. Please, come with me."

"But I haven't done anything wrong."

I put my hands on my hips. "Why would I assume you'd done something wrong?"

She lowered her eyes to the floor. "You told us to leave the new bottles alone, but I felt I needed to make sure all the pills were fully accounted for. After all, that's my job."

I nodded and said nothing as we made our way back to my office. Once she was seated in front of me, I said, "Regina, I know you have a problem and we need to get you some help. Okay?"

She held up her hands and pulled back. "Problem?! I don't have a problem. What are you talking about?"

Melva came into my office and stood behind her. "Here you go," she said laying the pills on my desk.

"What are these?" Regina said.

I picked a pill up and held it close to her. "These are fake Vicodins. You've replaced the real ones with fakes. I assume you've been ingesting them. The residents have been getting fakes. That's why you had to open the new bottle this morning. You needed to get a fresh supply."

She shook her head. "No, one of the other girls got into the cabinet with their key. Remember? They each have a key."

"I'm sorry, but they don't. They just think they do. They have fakes. You were the only one with a real key. Our company has been planning this little sting operation for weeks. We can't go on hurting the residents, preventing them from getting their prescribed medication. For crying out loud, you're a nurse! You of all people should understand."

Regina continued shaking her head. "You're wrong. You got it all wrong! I'm innocent. I don't have a problem. I don't even take Vicodin."

I smirked at her. "Okay, have it your way." Then I reached over, picked up the phone and dialed a number. "Billy please . . . Yes, I'll wait. . . . Hey Billy, we caught her . . . Yeah Regina, but she's denying it . . . Yes, sir. I'll call them as soon as I hang up. Thanks."

Regina shifted uncomfortably in her chair. "What did he say?"

"He told me to call the police and let them handle it. They'll test your urine and hair follicles today and review our evidence. They can decide if you have a problem or not." I picked up the phone and was about to dial when she stopped me.

"Wait! Okay, maybe I've taken a few Vicodin, but that doesn't mean I have a problem. I'll stop right now. No more problems with the pills or the residents. I swear."

I slid her a pen and a pad. "Write it all down and I'll talk to Billy. I'll see what I can do, but listen, no promises. Understand?"

She seemed relieved. "Yeah, I understand."

"But Regina, listen to me. It'd better be the truth."

She nodded and began writing. When she was done she handed me the pad to read. She admitted to *occasionally* taking a few pills and *sometimes* shorting the residents, but according to her the residents needed to be weaned off them anyway. It was a minimal confession, one she hoped would match up with what she thought the evidence was. I put the pad down, leaned forward in my chair and conjured up the meanest, nastiest face I could. "Look, I want you to hand in your keys right now! And any Vicodin or fake pills you have on you. I want you to empty your pockets and let me see them. Now!"

She'd never seen me like this and it obviously scared her. Immediately she put the keys on the desk and began emptying her pockets. Pills spilled everywhere. Most were Vicodin, but several were fakes. I collected them into a plastic baggie and locked it in my drawer.

"Now, I want you to go home and start researching some rehabs, ones for hydrocodone. Understand?"

"Yes, ma'am. I will."

"Good, because I need to talk to corporate and see what they want to do."

"Look, it won't happen again. I promise. Just give me another chance. Please!"

"You're dismissed. Melva, escort her outside."

Melva nodded and left my office with a hunched over Regina in front of her. Now I had to call both Billy and Syp to let them know what had happened. Two weeks later, Regina was long gone with a report made on her nursing license. She would eventually lose it and have to start a career in another industry. DADS (Department of Aging and Disability Services) was called again and advised of the matter. With Syp's help, we avoided any violations. Still, I knew no matter how knowledgeable or connected he was, we couldn't keep dodging these bullets forever. Eventually one would get us—*or me.*

I put Regina's file away and decided to walk around the facility to find some of these problems before they happened. I had to get ahead of all of this. My first stop was the back patio where I wanted to see if the folks at Warm Heart were causing more problems for our residents. Ten days ago one of our residents, Bennie Malone, had gotten into a tussle with one of their residents. They were standing at the fence jawing at each other when according to witnesses, Warm Heart's resident bully, Old Blackie, grabbed Bennie's shirt and ripped it. Bully Number Two, Red Man, was standing there urging Old Blackie on. When Bennie came back inside he was wound up, saying he was leaving our home. Even though he had some mental issues, the court system hadn't judged him incompetent, mainly because they didn't know about him. He'd already started packing by the time I reached his room. I called in several staff members to try and talk him out of it, but nursing homes aren't prisons. We can't hold anyone against their will. In ten minutes, he'd packed up everything, called a cab and walked out the front door.

An hour later I received a call from one of our competitors asking for the various numbers for Bennie's insurance policy and Medicaid/Medicare coverage. They told me was now living with them and they'd be transferring everything over. I was upset. Not only were we not gaining ground, we were losing it. Then, something else happened.

I received a call two days later from Syp telling me that Bennie had bitten off the finger of one of the nurses at his new home and they had called the police. Before the police could get there, he'd caught a cab and was cruising around town, looking for a new place to stay. Syp figured he might come back here. I thought that was unlikely, but I assured him I'd keep a sharp lookout. No sooner had I hung up than Melva appeared at my door.

"Hey Susan, guess what? We're not so bad after all. Guess who's back?"

"Who?" I said turning my body away, hoping not to hear the answer I dreaded.

"Bennie!"

"Oh crap!" I sprung to my feet. "Where is he?"

Melva's brow furrowed. "He's heading to his old room, the one he'd shared with Mr. Martinez. His bed is still available."

I jumped up and ran. "Follow me!" I got there just in time. Bennie was at the door talking to Mr. Martinez when I slowed up and said, "Hey Bennie. How are you doing?"

He spun around and said, "Oh, hi Ms. Hodges. I was thinking of coming back."

"You are?" I said happily. "Why, we're excited you're considering us. Perhaps I can offer you something more. Please, get your bag and come with me."

As we walked to the front lobby, he was smiling at the possibility of a private room or some other treasured amenity. Stopping him, I said, "Excuse me for one second." I grabbed Melva's arm hard, pulling her away from Bennie and whispered, "Call a cab right now. Hurry!"

She was completely taken off guard, but knew me well enough to follow orders. Turning back to Bennie, I said, "Please, let me show you something out front. I have a great idea."

He went outside with me, wearing the same large smile and waiting for the big surprise. I spent the next few minutes speaking double talk and acting like I was prepared to make him a huge offer when the cab drove up.

"C'mon over here, Bennie. I want to tell you something." I opened the door and said, "I have a surprise for you. Get in." Still smiling, he got in the backseat with his luggage on his lap and turned to me for the payoff. Whispering so cab driver couldn't hear, I said, "Hey I know you just bit off the finger of a nurse, so staying with us is a no-go. Please go somewhere else and don't come back." Then I jerked back, slammed the door shut and yelled, "Thanks and have a good trip, Mr. Malone!" The cab pulled away with his no-longer-smiling face plastered up against the window. I assumed the police would eventually catch up to him and let him join Wayne in prison, but I never heard what happened.

Now I had another problem. When Mr. Martinez saw Bennie leave in a cab, he didn't know Bennie had bitten off a finger. He assumed Bennie had found a better place, so he started talking about leaving too. Here I stood watching him pack.

"I'm going to leave, Ms. Hodges."

"Where are you going?" I asked, casually blocking the door.

"I don't know. I'm just going to leave. Okay?" He kept packing.

I called for help. "But you like it here. The meals are good, you have friends here and it's a nice place to stay."

"Look, Ms. Hodges. No offense, but I'm fifty-nine years old and I don't want to turn sixty in this ~~shithole~~. Okay?"

One of his favorite CNAs arrived. "Candy, Mr. Martinez is leaving. He likes you. What do you have to say about it?"

She leaned into his room and started talking sweetly to him. This went on for a few minutes until his bag was packed. Then she walked with him down the corridor, trying to talk him out of it. I tried to grab some of the residents to help, but they could care less. In fact, if I weren't careful they'd think about joining him. The last thing we needed was a mass exodus. Like a run on the bank, other homes had experienced them and there was no reason it couldn't happen here. If the residents believed there was a much better place out there, they'd leave and never return. Even if they died on the street, as tragic as that was, it meant we'd lost them. If we lost enough, eventually we'd close down and I could start looking for my second job in the nursing home industry.

I hung my head and went back inside.

"Sorry, Susan. I tried."

"It's not your fault. Bennie got to him. We lost him by a nose, or actually . . . a finger."

Candy grinned and walked away, leaving me in a bad mood. In two weeks I'd lost my director of nursing and two residents. As I sat pouting in my office, I had to admit it seemed like I was losing this battle. Try as I might, I just couldn't make this place livable—*or lovable*—a home where people wanted to stay. Perhaps I'd made a big mistake. Maybe I wasn't cut out to be an LNFA. Then my phone rang.

"Hello, Susan Hodges speaking."

"Hey this is Billy." Oh brother! Just what I needed.

"Uhh Billy, I need to tell you something."

"Whatever it is it can wait. Go look out front."

"Out front?"

"Just do it and come back."

I went to the lobby and looked out. There was a large group of elderly people standing together on the sidewalk, looking mostly afraid. I blinked twice to make sure I was seeing what I thought I was seeing. Sure enough, two of them were Blackie and Red Man. But instead of the bird-shooting and puffed out chests, they now sported hangdog expressions as they kicked at some pebbles. Were they coming to apologize?

"Hey Billy, what's this about? There are maybe a dozen or so people outside."

"Thirteen to be exact. They're from Warm Heart. They just closed their doors this morning.

"Are you serious?"

"Yeah, I'm serious. You've been needing more residents, right? Well, here they are. The state contacted me and gave me first shot at some of them. I took as many as they'd give me. Turns out thirteen is the magic number."

"B-but these people hate our home. They're not going to like it here."

"No, they *used* to hate the home on the other side of the fence. Now this is *their* home and maybe they'll show you the same loyalty they showed when they lived at Warm Heart."

I was stunned. Not only was I about to receive a flood of new residents, but Billy hadn't coughed once. I considered both of these developments a small miracle. Maybe things were looking up.

"Okay, I'll get right on it."

"Oh and Susan, they're each holding checks. Make sure you get those to the bank pronto, like today. Okay?"

"Yes, sir!" Now I was grinning.

"Go get 'em Susan. You can do it. I have faith in you." The coughing started just before he hung up. At least some things never change.

9

"Quiet, people! I need your attention!" The group settled down and stared curiously at me, whispering among themselves. A few minutes earlier I'd asked Melva to go through the home and gather up the staff for this impromptu meeting.

"Melva, is that all of them?"

"Yeah, that's it."

I cleared my throat. "Okay people, here's the news. The Warm Heart Nursing Home—the one directly behind us—has closed. The state is dividing up the residents and placing them in various nursing homes. We've been given thirteen and we need to get them in and process them fast."

Muttering broke out as curious looks turned into frowns. Several placed their hands on their hips. I could hear the voice of my assistant director of nursing above the others saying, "I have to get my nails done at three. I don't have time for this."

Someone else piped up. "Yeah, I've got a doctor's appointment. I have to leave at quitting time."

I found their attitude extremely disappointing. "Look, even though these folks are having their lives turned upside down, I promise I'll do my best to make sure you aren't inconvenienced one bit. We still have an hour to go before shift change and can get a lot done by then, so listen up."

I directed them to get all of the current residents into the dining room for teatime. I wanted coffee and fruit punch made, tea served, and cookies and snacks available. If they were allowed to roam around, they'd start interacting with the new arrivals—their hated rivals—and who knew what would happen? Having them all in one place would make it easier for us to control and prevent flare-ups. I also had the TV turned on and a video inserted so their attention would be directed away from the lobby. Then I made sure we scattered around crossword puzzles and word search books and anything else that might catch their attention. My activities director assured me she would keep them occupied.

While Melva was busy getting with the admissions director to create thirteen folders, I had the nurses set up medical supplies to be ready to examine any of the new residents who might have health problems. Then I ran into the kitchen and told Alisha to prepare a rolling cart of fruit punch and snacks to keep near the lobby. Reading my mind, Carlos brought in some foldout tables and chairs to set up near the reception desk where we were going to process them. Despite the initial resistance, the staff was digging in nicely for the coming onslaught.

I glanced at my watch and realized it'd been over ten minutes since I'd received the call from Billy. That meant those folks had been out there for who knows how long. At least the weather was pleasant. Still, it was time to welcome them home.

"Okay people, I'm bringing them in. Melva, get some more CNAs to help me."

I went outside and looked the group over. Most of them were staring at the pavement and crying. As I got closer, a few lifted their heads. "Hello, I'm Susan Hodges. I'm the administrator here. Welcome to the Jones-Simms Nursing Center."

"Move aside!" came a voice from the back. The crowd parted to reveal a woman rolling towards me in a wheelchair. I could see she hadn't been crying. "Are you the boss here?"

"No, all the residents that reside here are my bosses, every last one of them. I get paid to help them take care of things. What's your name?"

"I'm Gracie. But what I wanna know is, are we gonna get beat up for calling your place a ghetto and a crap heap?"

I smiled. "No, of course you won't. This is *your* place now. The residents here will be your friends."

"Yeah, yeah, yeah, that's all great, but Ed and Roadie here, they're pretty sure they're gonna get it."

I could tell she was referring to Red Man and Old Blackie. Both men were staring intently at their shoes.

"Trust me. You're all welcome here. Let's just go inside, get you checked in and find a good room for you. Okay?"

She looked around at the others and said, "C'mon gang, let's get it over with. We can't sleep out here." She wheeled herself forward and the rest of the group followed. A CNA and I opened the door and stood by as they filed past. The first thing they saw was the cart of goodies waiting for them. This stopped whatever crying was still going on and allowed them to focus on what was to come. When they all had something to eat and drink and were seated around the tables, we selected one of them and began the enrollment process. Meanwhile, one of the nurses went around checking their vitals to see if we had any problems and a CNA took a photo of each one. I could tell that most of them were traumatized. They'd been so familiar with Warm Heart, its residents, staff, and routine. Then, just like that, it was ripped away and they were sent to the place they despised most of all. It had to be rough.

After each one was processed they were led them down the hall to select a room. Before my staff's shift ended, amazingly, we were almost done. Old Blackie and Red Man wanted to room together so we accommodated them. I could see they were no longer the mean bullies on the other side of the fence. Now, they looked like children who knew they'd been caught doing something wrong and were awaiting their punishment. But there was something more. They were very afraid. Our staff couldn't be everywhere every second of every day. They had to know this. Also, some of the men in the home were in their fifties and sixties—still able to cause some harm. Yet I hoped that by letting the new arrivals stay together it would help them protect each other. Of course, I was also determined to let nothing happen to them. I was the one who'd be hammered if anything went wrong.

I noticed Gracie was hanging around two others. They were the last three to be processed. While my staff raced through the paperwork, Gracie rolled over to me.

"Hey Administrator, Dale has a question for you." She motioned for the woman to come over.

"Are you Dale?" I asked.

"Yes, and that's Ari." She was referring to the man still seated at the table. "We were both wondering about what you said, about you working for us. Is that really true?"

"Of course. You have rights that are legislated by the state of Texas. It's my job to make sure you fully enjoy those rights. When you all get settled and come to dinner, I'll read those rights to you. I'll even give you a copy."

"Really?" Her eyes were wide and bright.

"Yes, really. Has no one ever gone over them with you before?"

"No, they haven't. Oh gosh, I can't wait."

"Okay, now go along with this nice nurse. She'll help you find a comfortable room and get you all fixed up."

Before she turned to leave, she grabbed my hand and shook it. "Thank you so very much."

"That's what I'm here for Dale."

As she left my office and walked down the hall, Melva came up to me. "That does it. They're all processed. We still need to do more work, but this should be enough to get them going."

"Did you hear what she just told me?"

"Yes, I did. What kind of place do you think that was over there?"

"I don't know, but not going over their rights is a huge violation. Let's go to my office and see what we have."

Once we were in my office, Melva handed me the files. I made some notes and set the last one on the stack. That's when my assistant director of nursing came in and gave me the short version. "Susan, I can't say for sure, but it looks like most of these people can be worked up to the point of getting back into a more independent facility. They don't need a field nursing facility like ours. Four of them look like they could leave right now. With proper medication and social programs, another four could probably leave in a few weeks and maybe a couple more in a month or two. However, I'm pretty sure the last three will have to stay."

"Yes," I said. "I was just looking over their files. The lady in the wheelchair, Gracie, looks like she'll be with us permanently unless we have a relative who can take care of her. Dale looks pretty frail and Ari seems to have some mental issues. Still, we'll have Dr. Lowery come in and do a full workup. He'll let us know."

The nurse nodded and left to go to her nail appointment. When the door closed, I turned to Melva. "It looks like none of them have high RUG rates, do they?"

"Nope. The last three need the most care, but they're pretty much walkie-talkies. We won't need to provide them a lot of services. But I do have good news. Most of the folks have huge checks. Here, look at what they came with."

I stared at the figures. "What?! $35,000. $28,000. That's crazy! At least the owner didn't steal it, like so many do."

"That's for sure. Normally the owner would've absconded and used it to hire lawyers to keep the prison years down. But this one appears to have simply put all their social security checks into a big pile and cut off access to it by the resident. The last three each have over $40,000. That'll pay us for quite some time. Unfortunately, they're all over the $2,000 Medicaid threshold. I'm going to call the state and tell them about it—I'm sure they didn't know. This will cause a Medicaid denial which means we'll have to start all over again to get them approved and the money flowing."

That gave me heartburn just thinking about it. "Call them right away and tell them what we have. We need to figure out something fast. And get those armbands made and on them. No sense in having them wander around this fine neighborhood and get lost."

"Or shot! I'll get on it."

We left my office and I went to thank the kitchen staff. "Alisha, you did a wonderful job. That cart worked perfectly. Now please do one more good deed for me: have a nice dinner ready, especially since they'll all be together."

"Okay. I'm going to stay late and help my second shift do it right. I heard the word's already spread about the newcomers and a great meal might calm everyone down."

"Word's spread?" This spiked my heartburn. "What did you hear?"

"Several residents were talking about kicking them out. You're going to have your work cut out for you."

"Thanks for the info. I'd better make my rounds and head off any problems."

I walked through the halls and found three residents standing at the entrance to Old Blackie's and Big Red's room. They were really going at it, yet neither newcomer was responding. They just stood there, taking it.

"Hey, break it up!" I said. "These are new residents and they're now our friends. If you can't say anything nice, go away and leave them alone." They didn't move. "Now! I mean it!" They'd never heard me yell before. It did the trick.

I poked my head in. "Sorry gentlemen. You tell me or one of the staff if this happens again. We'll take care of them, even if we have to call the police."

They nodded and said nothing. I walked away knowing this was going to be a recurring problem. I needed to figure a way to head it off.

By dinnertime I'd formulated a strategy. The first part involved their names. I worked with one of the CNAs to get their names up on each room so they looked like any other resident. I wanted everyone to see that they were now part of the home and not some temporary visitor to chase away. I also had one more trick up my sleeve.

When all the residents were seated, both old and new, I noticed the new ones were sitting in a cluster together. This wasn't what I wanted yet it was so predictable. I stood up and clapped my hands. "Ladies and gentlemen, we have some wonderful new people who've joined us today." Several residents frowned and smirked. "Before we serve the food, I want to take this opportunity to read you your rights as a resident here. I know you all have a copy, but I want the new folks to hear them. So, let's begin." More grumbling.

I took my time and slowly went through all twenty-four rights. (My current residents barely paid attention; they heard them all the time.) I occasionally looked up to see Gracie, Dale and Ari all staring intently, soaking up every word. When I was done, I had thirteen copies distributed to the newcomers and signaled for dinner to begin.

Like all the meals before, the plastic trays were served out. Our meal service resembled lunches served in a school cafeteria. Or a prison. Each person had both a preordained type and quantity of food unceremoniously plopped down on their tray. Next, we gave them a paper napkin rolled around a fork, knife and a spoon. Tiny milk and juice cartons were handed out and the residents dug in. They were so conditioned to eating at a certain time that my five-minute delay had made them very hungry. They were barely looking up from their trays.

Most of them were done within twenty minutes. Once again I rose and said, "Listen up folks. I think it's time for you to hold a resident's counsel and discuss any issues you might be having. Who's going to second that motion?" Technically it wasn't proper for me to move for a meeting, but no one was complaining. Mr. G, as we called him, raised his hand. "Good. Can I please have the officers come up here and run the council?"

Three residents made their way to the podium.

"As you know, no staff or outsiders are allowed to be present during your council without permission. Madame President, I'd like to remain along with my staff to answer any questions you may have about our new residents. May we remain?"

The president looked at the other officers and shrugged. "Sure, I guess." Then she turned to the residents. "Okay, who wants to start?"

Mr. G yelled out. "These bastards need to go. Now!"

"Yeah," another resident yelled. "I second the motion."

The president announced, "All those in favor of kicking out the newcomers, raise your hands." I could see it was a clear majority. Just what I was afraid of. She smiled at me and said, "Madame Administrator, will you please remove them?"

"May I speak first?"

She shrugged her shoulders. "It won't make no difference, but go ahead."

I cleared my throat. "Thank you Madame President and duly elected officers of the Jones-Simms Nursing Center. First, I hear your request loud and clear and will make it happen right away. Next, I want to say what a privilege it's been to serve you. I'm going to miss all of you. Now, where do you folks want to go? Which homeless shelter? Mr. G, there's one downtown. Can I get the bus to take you there tomorrow?"

"What?!" he yelled out. "I'm not going to no homeless shelter! These losers are the ones that are leaving."

"Yes Mr. G, they're leaving. That's been decided. And you'll be leaving too. Actually, all of you will. I need you to start packing tonight so we can drop you off to where you want to go."

The residents glanced around in confusion. "What?" the president said. "What are you talking about?"

"I'm talking about the sad truth. All thirteen newcomers brought checks with them. Large checks. I'm prohibited from telling you how much, but they're enough to keep us going for a long time. You all know we're hurting financially and you know this is a for-profit venture, yet most of you have been costing us money, not making us money. These thirteen would not only help keep us afloat, but they would also put us in the black. Now that they're being kicked out, their money will leave with them. That means we'll have to close down which means there will be no home for you to stay in. So by tomorrow you'd better have your stuff packed and ready to go. We can serve you breakfast, but then you'll have to be on your way. A few of you can be admitted to the hospital, but most of you will be out on the street. If you don't select a place, we'll push you out to where these newcomers were standing this morning. I'm going to leave now and start calling the shelters to see who can take you. I'll post a list on the bulletin board before I leave tonight for you to look at. Let the staff know which one you want to be dropped off at. I want each of you to know that I've truly enjoyed working for all of you. Goodbye."

With that I turned my back on them, went to my office and waited. Sure enough, ten minutes later I heard several people making a commotion outside my office. I picked up the phone and talked into it as they opened my door without knocking. "Yes ma'am. They can sleep in the open air. At least it's better than nothing. Thank you." I hung up the phone. "Can I help you folks?"

The president shuffled in. "Yes, uhh, we've reconsidered and voted to let them stay. But, we're going to hold a meeting next week in case we change our minds."

"We'll let you know," the vice-president added.

"Oh, that's wonderful!" I said clapping my hands. "Thank you for your generous spirit. You are truly kind. I don't have to look for a new job."

They grumbled and slinked away. With that the Warm Heart rivals were now assimilated into the Jones-Simms family.

The next morning I was briefed on how the night had gone while I was away. There'd been a few mouthy exchanges, but everything had stopped once they'd gone to bed. The staff felt confident the worst was behind us. As soon as my briefing ended, Dale came to the door.

"Ms. Hodges, may I speak to you?"

"Come in. And please call me Susan." I pulled out a chair for her as she limped in. "Here, have a seat. What can I do for you?"

She took a seat and rubbed her hands nervously. "Well, I read over my rights and was wondering if you could find out some things for me. Maybe help me."

"Absolutely. Like I said, I work for you. But I don't have your folder and medical records yet. We're supposed to get all the files from the owner of Warm Heart this afternoon. Until then, I won't know much."

"I understand, but I'm not looking for medical information. I need help getting out of this mess."

I leaned forward in my chair. "What mess are you in?"

"A legal mess, and that's the worst kind."

I nodded. "That's for sure. Why don't you tell me all about it and I'll see what I can do." I pulled out a pad to take notes having no idea that what she would tell me would begin to change my life forever.

Dale Waterson was born in St. Louis as an only child. She'd gone to college and earned a two-year degree in accounting. Upon graduation, she'd started a business—an antique store—a rarity for a woman back then. She soon met Brad, a man who took her boating on their first date. Having spent a lot of time with her father on his sailboat, she loved boating. She knew instantly he was the one. They got married and had a daughter named Brooke. Besides raising Brooke, she wrote to her congressman and senators about important issues. Her favorite quote was "The name American must always exalt pride," by President George Washington, March 1797. These words were ones she felt described her very essence. (The quote was also a favorite of Ari). Dale was very active in the community and looked after her neighbors. As I listened and watched, she was like that Aunt Bee character on *The Andy Griffith Show*, though much thinner. So far, it was a fairly typical life.

As she got older her husband Brad, who had been in the Air Force for thirty-one years, got sick. He was admitted to the VA and died of an infection at the age of sixty-one. That left Dale alone with her daughter. Unfortunately, she and her daughter didn't get along. Brooke liked the handouts of money she was getting from her parents and when Dale stopped those, the relationship turned sour. At least Dale had her antique store in Fort Worth to give her purpose.

One day some antiques fell over and injured Dale's right leg, crushing her foot. She was taken to the hospital and from then on walked with a limp. She was also suffering from a curvature of the spine and slumped over a lot. This made her look older than she really was. But she'd persevered through it all into her sixties and then into her seventies. By this time, her daughter Brooke was needing more money. Dale refused. Then one day she went to bed and life as she knew it disappeared forever.

Initially, she wasn't completely sure what had happened, but eventually pieced most of it together. When she didn't come into work for three days, an employee at the store called one of Dale's neighbors to check in on her. When they knocked, no one answered. They immediately called the police, who broke in. They found Dale in her bedroom, wedged between her bed and a wall. It appeared she'd rolled over and, lacking strength, slipped down, becoming hopelessly trapped. She was dehydrated and almost dead. They rushed her to the hospital where doctors worked hard to bring her back to health. This took over two weeks. It was when she was well enough to leave that she received the shock of her life. She was served with papers saying that she'd been judged incompetent and was now under the control of the court and two court-appointed guardians: a strange lawyer and her daughter Brooke. She was stunned. She hadn't even gone to court. How could this be?

The next day the court appointed guardian/lawyer came by to explain everything to her. While she was in the hospital, Brooke had hired a lawyer who brought in a doctor to examine her in the hospital. Since she was still out of it, she was deemed incoherent. Before the first week was up, a judge had declared her incompetent and made Brooke and the court-appointed lawyer her guardians. The minute the paperwork was signed, they began liquidating her antique store, selling off everything that wasn't nailed down. They also liquated her bank and retirement accounts, putting all her assets into a new bank account—one the lawyer controlled. They were going to use the money to place her in a nice, comfortable nursing home, one she would be very happy in. She tried to protest to the lawyer, but he smiled and told the CNA to take her away. So it was a complete shock to not only be in custody, but to be driven to a nursing home located in the Red Nine area. The moment she walked in, she knew it was a complete dump—certainly way below what she could afford. It didn't take her long to realize what was happening. She'd been taken to a cheap place to die so others could enjoy her life savings.

After her arrival, she discovered the doctor had prescribed drugs that essentially made her a walking zombie. Slowly but surely she used her infectious personality to avoid taking the drugs and get her mind clear. The nurses and CNAs of Warm Heart had no problem palming her meds and selling them on the street later. Or using the pills themselves. She also told me how their residents and ours had sold and swapped drugs over the fence. I was disgusted but not surprised.

By the time she got her mind free of the meds, months had ticked by. She discovered that with the lawyer's permission, Brooke had already spent a lot of the funds—over $1 million—and in two years had effectively bankrupted her. With no money to pay for her care, Warm Heart applied for Medicaid and kept her social security checks. When she was approved, they added the Medicaid reimbursement to her social security checks to pay for the entire cost of her stay.

Now she was eighty-one years old and five years of her life had evaporated. Everything was gone. She had been robbed blind and wanted to get out of this trap. Not long before, she'd demanded her court-appointed lawyer come visit her. He did and that was the last time he ever came back. In fact, he instructed his staff to stop taking her calls because she was calling too much, spouting the same 'conspiracy' nonsense. All she really wanted was an accounting of where all her money went. When she finally got one, it showed all the money went to both the lawyer and Brooke. Essentially, Brooke had found a neat way to receive all of her inheritance while Dale was still alive. Of course, the lawyers got a fat percentage too. According to her, she was the victim of a crime, yet she was the one in prison.

At the end of her story she asked me to contact both her court-appointed lawyer and Brooke and have them both come and visit. Then, she wanted to use some of the surplus money she'd brought over from Warm Heart to hire a different lawyer and bust her out. I made detailed notes of all this. Normally, I would've thought it was the ramblings of a demented mind. Yet my interactions with her told me she was not only sane, but also completely competent. Her story was too clear. I promised I'd look into it and would keep her updated, after I got her files. She understood that and we shook hands as she left.

Several hours later I received the files from Warm Heart. I anxiously thumbed through the stack looking for Dale's file. When I found it, there was nothing to contradict anything she had told me. But as I got to the financial page, I saw it there in black and white. At the bottom of a long list of medical expenses was this simple line: Monthly Court-Appointed Guardian Fee – $45.00.

10

I thought hard about Dale's situation. Seeing that $45 charge was beginning to open my eyes to all that Syp had told me. As the LNFA, I'm responsible for a lot of things but I'm not a lawyer. I'm not required to untangle a legal mess or go to court for someone. Yet I'm also a human being with feelings, morals and ethics. If someone's drowning, I'm not the type who can simply stand by and watch. That, more than anything else, is why I picked up the phone and called Dale's lawyer. The secretary put me right through.

"Yes, what is it?" he said.

"Hi, I'm Susan Hodges, the administrator at Jones-Simms Nursing Center. I wanted to let you know your client Dale Waterson has been transferred to our home. The home she was staying in—Warm Heart—closed down. The state shifted her here, which is actually located right behind Warm Heart. I just received the file and wanted to give you the address."

I could hear him shuffling some paper around. "Go ahead," he said in the same hurried tone he'd answered the phone with.

After I gave it to him I could tell he was about to hang up so I blurted out, "Wait! Don't you want to know how she's doing?"

"No, not really. I've had a lot of problems with her. I don't need her calling my office every day bothering the staff. Please make sure that doesn't happen, okay?"

"But she's your client. Don't you have a fiduciary duty to make sure she's taken care of?"

"Look," he said, his voice growing louder, "until you get a law degree, don't lecture me on what my duties are. Or I'll just have the judge issue an order bringing you into court so you can tell him about his duties. Understand?"

I was stunned how this was lining up perfectly with what Dale had told me. Then he continued. "And for your information, she's obsessed with some wild conspiracy theory. She's crazy. You have the records, so you know. Now listen clearly, I can't deal with her and I don't have to. I report to the judge. That's who I work for."

"But sir, I thought you work for Dale."

"We're done here. Goodbye and don't call again." *Click.*

I set the phone down and leaned back in my chair. Of course he may be right—Dale could be crazy. Many of our residents had dementia or other mental issues. Yet she seemed so clear and lucid. Maybe she was fooling me. Or maybe she was telling the truth. I looked at the file again and found her daughter's phone number. After four rings, I heard the sound that told me she was clicking over from another call. "Hello," she said.

"Is Brooke available?"

"This is Brooke. Who's this?" Her attitude burned my ears, which was odd. I'd said only three words and already she was upset. I suspected it was the lawyer on the other line and he'd just filled her in on my call.

"Hi, I'm Susan Hodges, the administrator at Jones-Simms Nursing Center. I wanted to let you know your mother Dale has been transferred to our home."

"Yeah, okay. Is there anything else I can do for you?"

Now it was clear she'd just been talking to the lawyer—she was ready to hang up before she even got our contact information.

"Do you want to know how your mother is doing?"

"Look, my mother is a bitter woman. She's very negative. I did what was best for her but she rejected everything. Now she hates me and keeps trotting out this ridiculous conspiracy theory. I'm exhaust-ed dealing with her, so now it's your turn. Okay?"

"Okay. But don't you want to visit her? You're her only relative, her only child. She has no one else."

"No. Besides, she has you now." *Click.*

This was crazy. Sure, I'd seen relatives who'd fought with an el-derly person trying to get them the care they actually needed. It was a tough struggle, one that usually left the family scarred. It was possible Brooke had been through all that. Then again, it was also possible Dale was telling the truth. In fact, it was looking more and more like she was. And now she wanted me to start calling lawyers for her. I was thinking about how to go about it when Melva came bursting into my office.

"Well, I worked everything out with the state! They've reviewed the files and said that three of them should stay with us. Right now they're working to get the other ten placed in assisted living centers or with relatives. We think with APS's help (Adult Protective Services) they can be supplemented with Meals on Wheels and other services to keep them out of our home. Tomorrow they're having all of their personal stuff brought over from Warm Heart. Then the state is go-ing to take the money from the three who are staying long term and go on a spending spree. DADS is going to buy nice beds, furniture and new clothes for each one of them. Have you ever heard of such a thing?"

"No, I haven't."

"Me neither. And by the end of the week they'll have the accounts back under $2,000 so when our reports are due it'll show they're all in compliance. The ones who'll be leaving soon will even have a surplus once we're paid. What do you think about that?"

"I like it. At least we get to keep three. That'll make a nice dent in our vacancies. Which ones are they?"

"The ones we talked about—Ari, Dale and Gracie—'The Almond Joys' as the staff are calling them. They have a sweet nature, are a joy to be around, and their sense of humor is whimsical and sometimes nutty. 'The Almond Joys' seems to fit them. They pretty much hang together, especially Dale and Ari. They seem to need each other."

I thumbed through the list of names. "Do you know how many of the thirteen are on that guardianship program from the probate court?"

"The three who are staying. Why?"

What a nice coincidence, I thought. I decided to say nothing more until I could sort all of this out. "Okay. Anything else?"

"That CNA we just hired, the one who came over from Warm Heart? She said the owner was basically honest but in over her head. The direct deposits piled up and she lost all the financial control. She also took way too many charity cases. She didn't have a competent person working to get the cases approved by Medicaid, so she lost tons of money. She also said that the Almond Joys were running the joint, making it a fun place to work at. She's happy to be with them again. They seem to like her too. It's helped ease the transition."

"If the Almond Joys are running the place, does that mean I'll be out of a job?" I asked, smiling.

"We'll see. I'm sure she's exaggerating. But I've spent some time with them and they're pretty endearing. They're making it a point to get around and meet all the residents. It's fun to watch."

"Then it sounds like we're keeping the right three."

After Melva left, I realized that with the state going on a spending spree, Dale's account would drop to less than $2,000. That would make it difficult to hire a lawyer to help her. I would need to find a lawyer to work on the cheap or I'd have to first do the initial legwork on her allegations and then look for a free lawyer once I had a solid case, if such a human being existed. Regardless, I'd have to tell her about my two calls.

Before I could get to Dale though, Gracie came banging into my office with her wheelchair. "Hey Administrator, we've got a problem!"

"What is it?" I asked, taking a deep breath.

"You need to come and see."

Before I could answer she spun herself around and rolled away. I followed her down the hall, watching how fast she could roll. In no time she'd reached a room two doors down from where she was staying with Dale. I walked in to find both Dale and Ari already there. All three were gathered around the occupant of the bed and staring at me.

"What seems to be the problem here?"

"He can't move," Gracie said. "We can't let him live like this. We have to help him."

The 'him' they were referring to was Felipe, a forty-five-year-old invalid who was here when I started. "Felipe, do you feel like answering their questions?"

"Yeah, I guess."

Dale leaned over the bed and looked at his face. "Can you move your head to see us?"

Staring straight up to the ceiling, he said, "No. I'm paralyzed from the shoulders down."

"Oh my goodness! How long have you been here?"

"Six years."

Dale glanced over at Ari and Gracie. "How did this happen?"

Felipe paused for a moment. "It was a failed suicide."

Dale jerked away and pressed her hands to her face. "What?!"

"Yeah, I tried to hang myself and fell. All I did was break my neck, but it didn't take my life."

"Oh, my goodness." She was a little stunned, so Gracie rolled in closer.

"Is there anything you like? Anything we can do for you?"

Felipe smiled. "Yeah, I like jelly beans. Sometimes the nurses will put a jellybean in my mouth and let me enjoy it. Green and turquoise are my favorites. I like the white ones too. But they don't normally have jelly beans here, just on special occasions."

"Then guess what? We're going to start visiting you and feeding you jelly beans. My name is Gracie. I'm in a wheelchair and believe me, if I could get out of this chair I'd let you see my face. Dale was the first one who talked to you and Ari is with us, too. Say something, Ari."

"A brave man is a worthy man."

"He talks mostly with quotations. It helps keep his mind sharp."

Felipe smiled. "Okay. Nice to meet all of you. I hope you come and visit more often."

"We'll do more than that. You'll see."

With that, the Almond Joys made their way outside and down the hall, out of Felipe's hearing. Gracie spoke first. "Administrator, we're going to have to make some changes."

It looked like the CNA we hired from Warm Heart was right. "What changes do you propose?"

Before she could tell me, Dale stepped in. "How cruel is that?"

"What?" I said with an attitude. "What do you mean 'how cruel is that'?"

"Well, he's lying in a bed on his back and he can talk to you, but he can't move."

"Yes, that's all true. So?"

"What do you do with him? I mean, how does his life go on? I can't imagine being like that. He's got to be bored out of his mind."

"We have an activity director . . ."

Dale put her hands on her hips. "So?"

"She takes a boombox and sets it up with some music. Then she takes stuff that smells good and makes his room nice. After the music is over, she comes back and gets the box."

Dale frowned. "Are you kidding me? That's all you do for this man?"

I wanted to say, "No, that's not all we do for him. He's required to be in a semi-private room with someone else, but we let him have a private room." Instead, I kept quiet. Still, I wasn't used to being dressed down by residents like this and was about to mention it when she added, "That's awful! It's just awful!"

I glared at her. "Do you think you can do better?"

"We'll figure something out and let you know."

Ari walked up to me and said, "Where there's a will there's a way!"

The Almond Joys left me standing in the hall without feeling much joy. I glanced at my watch and headed back to my office. I had several candidates coming in for the director of nursing position and wanted to be ready for them. These three would have to wait.

Three days later a lot had changed. First, I'd hired Cayla, a DON to replace Regina. She seemed both caring and competent. She was going to review all of our nursing staff and make sure they followed the rules and were performing proper medicine. With that item crossed off my list, I had a talk with Dale. She wasn't surprised about my conversations with either her lawyer or her daughter. When I told her about the money being drawn down by the state, her eyes began to water. "Maybe with the $2,000 I can find a lawyer to look into it."

"Yes," I said, knowing the odds weren't good. "We might also find a lawyer to do it for free if we can get some more information. I have a few sources and I'll start digging into it, if you'll let me."

"Oh yes, please do. I hope to God you find something."

When she left, I said a prayer for God to open my eyes to anything I needed to know. I also added that request to my morning prayers at the back door before the start of each day. I knew all things were possible with God.

Next up was the state. Their representatives had come to our home, interviewed the Almond Joys and left with a long list of stuff to buy. When they returned, the three residents had nice new beds and mattresses. They also purchased a unique dresser for each one and stuffed it with new clothes, underwear, socks and shoes. It was like Christmas. Then I discovered something incredible: they had asked the state to purchase several items that weren't for themselves. One item was several large bags of jellybeans. As soon as they opened the bags, they spent time picking out the green and turquoise beans and went to Felipe's room to feed him some. But the biggest shock was the used overhead projector. I couldn't understand why they'd purchased that—until I saw their plan.

Once Carlos had fetched them an extension cord they set it up in Felipe's room and turned the triangle lens up towards the ceiling. Both Dale and Gracie started out with shadows created by their hands. They soon moved up to more sophisticated displays. Using sand, they were able to tell a story by drawing palm trees and an ocean. They created a little boat coming towards the island and before I knew it, they were professionals. I'd never seen Felipe so entertained. He just lay there staring up at the ceiling and watching them tell this wonderful story. It was simply amazing. Before long, nurses and CNAs were coming in to see and hear the stories too. Felipe's room was always packed.

This went on for several days in a row and showed no signs of letting up. Of course, they also fed him jellybeans. I was sure there was no one else in Texas receiving this kind of attention. Little did I know that this was just the beginning. These three characters had told me there was no reason this home couldn't be a wonderful and enjoyable place to live. They knew they were here for the long haul and decided to make the best of it. Now, all I had to do was sit back and enjoy the show.

11

It had been a few weeks since the Almond Joys had made Felipe their personal mission. Each day they spent a lot of time entertaining him. Whenever they put on a show it seemed like a magnet, attracting staff and residents alike. One day while I was watching one of their stories, I stole a look at Felipe and saw tears trickling down his face. It wasn't that the story was particularly sad. It was just that these people really cared about him. If a person ever doubted there was any hope for humanity, one session in Felipe's room would've set them straight.

That afternoon Gracie came barging into my office, her wheelchair pushing my door open. "Administrator, we need a Geri chair."

"A what?"

"A Geri chair. You know, the kind that rolls around and leans back. We need it for Felipe."

I held up my hands. "I know what one is, but they cost a lot of money. We simply don't have room for that in the budget right now."

She smirked at me. "I figured you'd say that. If we get the government to give us the money, will you use it to buy one?"

"Gracie listen, the government looks for every way to avoid giving us money. So please don't get your hopes up. Besides, how do you plan on getting it?"

"We're gonna write to our elected officials and tell them about the situation. We can be persuasive when we have a good cause. And getting Felipe up and around is a good cause. Don't you agree?"

I nodded. "Of course it is. Let me know if I can help."

"Just make sure these letters get mailed, okay?"

"That's easy. I promise." She was backing herself out of my office when I stopped her. "Hey, can I talk to you about something?"

"Sure, what's up?"

I pulled out her folder; it was as thick as Dale's. "I've been looking through your records—especially your medical conditions—and as much as I love having you here, it just seems like we might be able to get you with a relative, if you have one available. How did you end up in a nursing facility anyway? Would you mind telling me?"

Gracie frowned. "Well, it's long story. Do you really want to hear it?"

"I have time. After all, this is what I do. Go ahead and tell me all you want to."

"Okay, but you asked for it."

I had asked for it and she told quite a story. Gracie was born in 1924 and had a brother twelve years older. Her parents did manual labor for jobs, yet wanted more for their daughter. Unfortunately, they had very little education and no money to make it happen. So they urged her to take a lot of trade classes in high school. She followed their advice but during her senior year she received a surprise: she was pregnant. The boy responsible married her, but left her just six months after Mae was born. Gracie never saw or heard from him again. She certainly never received any money from him.

Years later, Gracie decided to move on with her life and get a divorce, but between the court, the lawyer, and her difficulty paying the legal fees, the paperwork never came through. To this day she wasn't sure if she was married or not. That one relationship with a man had soured her so much that she never married again and rarely ever dated. Instead, she took care of Mae and loved on her like there was no tomorrow.

Mae, though, had her own problems. She was a slow learner with a low IQ. With Gracie's pushing, Mae took special education classes and graduated high school, but that didn't ensure a solid income. With Mae's issues, she could only hold down labor-intensive work. Gracie would have to support her.

Gracie said her first job became her life's profession—a short order cook. Since she was a hard worker and had the job down pat, she was never unemployed for long. As she said, "I could sling that hash." Without much income, she lived in rental homes all her life and drove unreliable vehicles. "I couldn't afford anything decent."

Like Dale, Gracie had been involved in her community. She had been a part of her neighborhood watch and got her name in the paper when she saw a man breaking into a house, called the police who caught him. She even kept the article framed in her house.

Gracie was also a family person. She and her brother had taken care of her mom and dad during their final years, never asking for anything in return. Once though, her mother gave her a very special gift: a locket with a diamond in the center. The diamond was very tiny, but it was real. Gracie was extremely proud of it—it was truly precious to her. Over the years the chain became worn and eventually broke into pieces. To replace it Gracie found some very thin, yet strong twine. She painted it gold and put four separate hard knots in it, so if one gave way the others would hold. If one didn't look too close, it resembled a gold chain. Eventually, it would be passed down to Mae, whom she knew would love and cherish it as much as she did.

Over the years, the movements needed for a short order cook wreaked havoc on her joints, especially her hips. The standing didn't help either. She adjusted by using sliding stools and a cane to get the job done. Finally, though, she gave up and retired. Of course, retirement was more of a word than a reality since she had no money saved up; she had no assets other than a cheap car and a bit of furniture.

A year earlier Mae had met a boy who was also a slow learner. Mae worked at the Goodwill center getting donated items ready to sell. Wally, also challenged, rode with a truck driver unloading the donated items. They met and sparks flew. The young couple was apparently smart enough to figure out a few things because soon, Mae became pregnant and eventually had two children with Wally. They all lived with Gracie. With Gracie's social security check and their income, they were somehow able to make it.

As the years rolled by, Gracie transitioned to a wheelchair, however it wasn't easy seeing everything from four feet off the ground. Her wheelchair was used and rundown; she couldn't afford anything better.

When Gracie's brother died of a heart attack, he left everything to her. This amounted to over $50,000. It was the most money she'd ever seen. She spent some of it burying him next to their father. Their mother was on the other side, with a spot waiting for Gracie. She wasn't yet ready to go, but took comfort in knowing that someday she'd be lying next to her family, completing their little band.

Gracie spent the weekdays babysitting her grandchildren when they came home from school. One day, her oldest granddaughter, Mattie, was pushing her around in the wheelchair. Mattie couldn't see over the wheelchair, so Gracie was helping to steer. As they got closer to a cat that was sleeping on floor, Gracie told Mattie to stop. Mattie didn't seem to hear her. Gracie managed to apply the brakes, stopping just in time. Mattie, however, was unprepared and jammed her face into the handle of the wheelchair. In seconds the tears flowed and screams echoed down the hall. Gracie tried to help her, but the child ran to her room and cried. Several hours later Mae came home and found Mattie in her room. She had a red welt near her eye, but otherwise seemed fine. They had dinner and forgot all about it.

The next morning, Mattie came to breakfast with a nasty shiner on her cheek. She wasn't happy about it, but Mae insisted she go to school anyway. As soon as a teacher saw the injury, she called Child Protective Services (CPS) who examined Mattie and learned her grandmother had injured her. They made an unexpected visit to the home, where Gracie was wheeling around like normal. After seeing their living conditions and learning more about the IQs of Wally and Mae, the CPS caseworker called in Adult Protective Services (APS). That caseworker examined an uncooperative Gracie and discussed the situation with the CPS caseworker. Before the sun was down, Gracie was forcibly taken to a healthcare facility and the two grandkids were taken into protective custody. Mae and Wally were devastated.

One thing that didn't help was Gracie's colorful language, a product of working for and around men in cafés and restaurants. Cuss words often flew out of her mouth. "You're not taking my ass anywhere," she'd yell. Or, "I have rights, you piece of shit!" All this certainly didn't help her cause.

She was taken away and then examined by a doctor, who later testified that she was incompetent and needed help managing her affairs. He said it was best if the court could take jurisdiction over her. When the judge granted the motion finding her incompetent, Gracie let loose with her profanity, making matters even worse. She was later introduced to a man who said he was her guardian ad litem and would be taking care of her. However, his version of 'taking care of her' seemed to consist of spending most of his time going over her financial affairs and trying to understand what assets she owned. Within a few weeks he'd drained her bank account and sold her car and furniture. They even got rid of the framed newspaper article. When he came back to get information about her cemetery plot, she tried to physically attack him, but being in a wheelchair, she couldn't do much. A few days later she received a letter stating they had sold her plot. Now she was penniless and could qualify for Medicaid. That caused her to cry and cry. "I'll never be near my family again!" And to make matters worse, a stranger would be buried right next to her mother. It was too much to bear.

ie wrote to Mae, who was completely distraught. Mae was

ʒ in some government assisted living center for folks like

her, along with her boyfriend and the two children. The government took the majority of her and Wally's money. With the cost of the bus and the time it took to get to the Warm Heart Nursing Center, she could only visit about once every six weeks. It was all such a tragic end to a long road.

Gracie had cried many times over all of this. Even though Mae didn't have the mental ability to handle her affairs, they'd all been getting along fine. Now, she was helpless to stop the financial plundering and imprisonment she was experiencing. At the same time, she knew her years were limited. She could scream and cry every minute of every day or try to make the best out of it. So that's what she decided to do. "I'm not going to let those criminals steal my remaining years, too. They took everything else and they ain't getting that!"

The weight of what I heard was heavy. Once again I was seeing a few common threads running through some of the people in my care. I decided to probe a bit farther. "When you were at Warm Heart, did you pay a monthly fee of $45 to a court?"

"Maybe. I really don't know. We saw no money and had no way of spending any of it, even if she'd given it to us. I have no idea what money comes in for me. No idea at all."

"You won't find that happening here. We're available to give you an accounting any time. In fact, you now have a little less than $2,000 in your account while each month $45 goes to the court to take care of you."

"You mean to imprison me!"

"Well, whatever they're doing, they're taking the money out of your account. Whenever you want to go over it, see Melva and she'll show you the printout. We'll take you shopping every now and then or have someone go out and get whatever you want. Okay?"

"Okay. You're a pretty good deal, Administrator. I guess I'm lucky to have you."

"I prefer to say *blessed*."

"Hell, that's fine with me. Blessed."

We finished our conversation and I wished her well on getting the Geri chair. I knew there was a better chance of me making the Dallas Cowboys roster than seeing a Geri chair come rolling in, but who was I to rob her of hope. She'd been robbed enough already.

The next day was Friday. When the mail arrived I found two letters addressed to me personally. The first was from Red Man. He'd moved to an assisted living center that had more freedom than our place. He was extremely grateful for the help and overjoyed to be a few blocks from his family. The second letter was from Old Blackie. He first apologized for his terrible behavior and then thanked me several times. He'd landed with a nephew who had an extra room, and with the community help we found for him, he felt like he was free again. He couldn't thank me enough, especially since we could've treated him harshly. He said he'd never forget what I had done.

Of course, it wasn't just me. It was our entire team. Still, as an administrator I knew I had the power to make the lives entrusted to me miserable or wonderful. It was a big responsibility, yet one I relished. Sure, I wanted to make more money and I wanted our company to profit, but having my residents happy and content in their final years was worth far more.

As I set the letters down I remembered that I had another pleasant chore to do. I found Carlos and led him to my office. "Congratulations, Carlos. You've been voted Employee of the Year!"

He clapped his hands in excitement. "Wow! That's great. What do I get for that?"

"Well, you're going to get a pin to wear," I said with bubbling enthusiasm.

He seemed somewhat disappointed. "Okay, what else?"

"Uh, well you'll get a small plaque so you can show it off in your home."

He leaned forward. "Okay, anything else?"

I could see his initial excitement was dropping straight to the floor and knew this next item wouldn't bring it back up. "We'll post a plaque in the hall with your name on it."

"Gee, thanks," he said in a sarcastic tone.

"Oh wait, I forgot! You get your very own parking space. The one closest to the door. That's something!" I gave it one last hard sell, almost like he was getting a raise.

"Okay Susan, I get it," he said pushing back the chair and standing in front of me. "The joke's on me."

"What?! This isn't a joke. Why are saying that?"

A wry smile creased his face. "You know good and well I don't own a car. What am I going to park there, my tennis shoes?"

I checked my surprise. I'd completely forgotten. In fact, only Melva and I had cars. As such, there were always spaces available to park so really, even if he had a car it wouldn't have been anything at all.

"I'll tell you what, let me see what I can do. Okay?"

"Whatever. Is there anything else?"

"No," I said, as he walked out of my office. Then I added loudly, "Again, congratulations!" With his back to me he held up his hand as if to wave. Frankly, I was relieved to see all five fingers sticking up.

I knew he'd gotten a raw deal, but I also knew we didn't have the money in the budget for anything more. To fix this I reached into my own pocket and purchased $150 gift certificate from Wal-Mart. Then I called him in the next day and told him I'd buy his space from him. He smiled and accepted my offer. After that, I drove up to work each day and had two parking spots to choose from, along with the others that never held a car. At least my Employee of the Year was happy—*somewhat.*

It had been six weeks since the Almond Joys entered our facility. During that time, no one had visited them. I knew Dale wasn't likely to have anyone show up and I didn't know Ari's story yet, but I wondered about Gracie. Then, one day her daughter showed up and what a treat it was! Mae had taken the bus and come on a Tuesday morning for a three-hour visit. She and Gracie talked and talked. Dale and Ari joined in too. It was like Mae was related to all three of them. Gracie had no problems sharing her daughter and this was unusual. Residents rarely have visitors so when one finally does come, sharing them never happened. Yet that was the kind of person Gracie was. She was happy sharing everything.

One ritual I saw them go through was centered around the diamond necklace Gracie wore. As soon as Mae arrived, Gracie would take it off and let Mae wear it. Mae thought it was worth thousands of dollars and didn't seem to understand the painted twine was not actually gold. Mae put it around her neck and looked in the mirror like she was now rich. It was truly heartwarming to watch. Mae wore that necklace the entire visit, before carefully removing it and putting it back around Gracie's neck. "Until the next time," she said. Then Mae hugged Dale and Ari hard and gave one last hug to Gracie before leaving. Afterwards, all three Almond Joys found a spot to gather where they could discuss the visit. They went through any news Mae had brought and anything else they could remember. It was like watching three people pick a Thanksgiving turkey clean. By the time they were done, there was nothing left to discuss. That meant it was time for a nap.

After work that night it was time to get together with Vicki. We hadn't seen each other in ages. I was looking forward to getting caught up. We met at our usual restaurant and were two glasses of wine into our visit when she broke the news. "I caught my BOM stealing $20,000 from the residents' accounts. She was arrested and her lawyer cut a plea bargain. Now she's heading to prison."

"What?! I caught my DON stealing hydrocodone, but nothing like $20,000. That's terrible. Did you get the money back?"

"No," she said sipping on her wine. "But the state is on us to reimburse the accounts. Our lawyer is talking to them."

"How did you catch her?"

"Actually, a lady who works for the court inadvertently helped me find it. She works for a probate judge—they're the ones who take that $45 out of the residents' accounts. When she wasn't getting paid, she showed up pissed, demanding her money."

"What's her name?"

"Nala Stahl. They call her Nala the Wall. She's tough to deal with. Real tough. Believe me, don't cross her!"

This matched what Syp had told me. "How many residents do you have in that court program?"

"Fourteen, and it seems like they're adding more each week."

"Have any of your residents complained about it? The court fees and the guardianship program?"

"Yeah, probably over half. Some of them are definitely incompetent and need help managing their affairs. But the rest are fairly competent, at least to me. They do have their moments, though. Many of them complain that their stuff was taken and sold and that they were shipped off to a home against their will. Sometimes it's a lot of money we're talking about. Our home isn't like yours—some of the folks had over $100,000 in assets and others close to $1 million. Someone, I don't really know who, got a doctor to say they're incompetent. The judge signed the order, appointed a lawyer, and within weeks the life they knew was gone. These court people are so aggressive I sometimes think *they're* our clients, not the residents."

"Exactly! I have ten on the program and with your fourteen, that's twenty-four. That's over $1,000 a month and almost $13,000 a year. And that's just our two homes, not to mention whatever happened to their assets."

"But at least they're helping us fill up our homes. That counts for something, right?"

"No, not right! Do you think it's acceptable to take competent folks, shove some pills down their throats, and rip their lives away? That could happen to us, you know. We're not immune."

Vicki laughed. "Well, I have a long time to go before that happens to me."

I remained serious. "I don't. I'm almost sixty. They could zap me for looking at them the wrong way. I was told to stay out of it, but I'm not sure I can now."

Vicki grew serious. "Look, I met this Nala. Whoever told you to stay away, they're right. Stay away. These folks aren't messing around. They kept telling me, 'You're violating a court order. Do you want to go to jail? Do you want to see the judge?' I was lucky to drive home in my own car and not a squad car. They act like they have God Himself behind them. Believe me, they're ten times worse than the state."

I listened to everything and filed it all away. I still had doubts that it was as bad as everyone was saying, but the doubts were rapidly shrinking. I also knew my personality was not one to walk away from anything like this. That meant I could be on a collision course with something big and nasty.

After dinner I went home, and as usual, set my cell phone next to my bed. Unfortunately, I'd turned off the sound during my dinner with Vicki and failed to turn it back on. That's why, when I sat down for breakfast and casually checked my phone, I almost had a panic attack. There were twenty-six messages from the home. I knew right away something extremely bad had happened.

I took a pad and began listening to the messages. Sure enough it was bad.

12

By the time I'd finished all the messages my blood pressure was through the roof, but at least I had the gist of it. In the middle of the night, Liddy, one of our CNAs, was moving Felipe so she could change the sheets. Felipe was heavy—what we call dead weight. Because he was paralyzed he couldn't help anyone who was lifting him so we had to use the Hoyer lift. The Hoyer lift has a fabric support that goes under the resident and attaches to a crane, which lifts him up. Everything is motorized and safe so as long as the CNA places the fabric in the proper location. According to Liddy, she was lifting Felipe when the Hoyer lift jerked unexpectedly and rolled him against the metal side-railing on his bed. This railing is not designed to support dead weight like Felipe's; it's designed for people to use when they are pushing the bed around. The Hoyer lift shifted his weight against the railing the bolts holding it gave way, dumping him on the floor. The CNA then panicked (along with everyone else on duty). Here was a quadriplegic, injured and bleeding profusely all over the floor.

An ambulance rushed him to the hospital where they took him directly into surgery. When I listened to the last message, I knew that there was nothing I could do at this point, so I finished what

I could of my breakfast and drove to work with a good deal of trepidation.

When I arrived, I paused at the back door and said my morning prayer, "Dear Lord, I need your help getting through this day. Please watch over Felipe and heal him. Bring him back to us safe and healthy. Amen."

I'd just put my things on my desk when Cayla, the new DON, came into my office to brief me on everything. "Susan, I called the hospital and got an update. He has a broken nose, a fractured eye socket, a cut over his eyebrow, a chip in the right side of his jaw and a smaller chip on his left side. Two teeth are loose, but it looks like they'll stay in place. There doesn't appear to be any spinal injury, thank God. Right now he's out of surgery and in recovery."

"That's pretty bad, but I was expecting much worse. Have we notified his family?"

"Yes. They're going by the hospital this afternoon to see him, once he's awake."

I let out a deep breath. "All right. Let me call DADS and get the reports going. This is going to be a huge boondoggle for sure."

"Oh and one more thing. I talked with Liddy before she went off shift. She's freaking out. She keeps switching between wondering if she killed Felipe or if she's going to get fired. She's supporting four kids all on her own and needs this job. She kept saying it was the machine, it was the bed, it wasn't her fault. I told her to take some time off but we'd probably need her to talk to the state if they requested it."

"Well, she might have to get fired. I don't know yet. Let's see how the investigation goes. Right now I need to make some calls so let me get to it."

"Okay." She opened my door to leave and before she could close it the Almond Joys barged in.

I interrupted them before they got all of the way in. "I've got my hands full right now. I don't have time for whatever you have there. So please, just let me . . ."

"Wait!" Dale said. "We've already done a lot of work for you."

"Work? What are you talking about?"

Dale handed me a leaf of papers. "We started early and worked through the night to make sure we could get as many as we could. You'll see that there are fourteen. All of them indicate the same thing. It was an accident." She thrust the papers at my chest. I fanned them out and discovered they were actual witness statements written by the residents about the incident.

I fumbled for the right words. "It looks like Jones-Simms has some seasoned detectives residing here. I can see from these reports that you folks heard about this incident, huh?"

Gracie spoke up. "Heard about it? We saw it and it was pretty fucked up! One of the nastiest, disgusting, regurgitating things I've ever seen. I thought he was dead. Good thing I was wrong."

Ari stepped in front of Gracie. "I am here to set the record straight."

Dale spoke up again. "Now honey, you're only one person and we're three. Let us help you with this. I guarantee all three of us are, without a doubt, the nosiest people in this home. We can get to the bottom of anything."

I thought about what my response should be. I didn't want them disrupting the place with more detective work, yet I could tell they really wanted to help. I decided to be diplomatic. "You three have done a great job. Let me review all these statements and see what else I need. Just hold off until I let you know, okay?"

"Okay, boss," Gracie said. "C'mon gang. Let's get moving and let the administrator do her job."

As they left, Ari said, "The truth shall set you free. John 8:32."

Dale patted him on the shoulder. "Nicely said, Ari."

I smiled and shook my head as they walked out. Every day was an adventure with them.

With my office free I dialed up Billy. Then Syp. Once again Syp had specific instructions on how to handle the state. Next I notified the state about the incident. They responded by saying an investigator would be coming out and sure enough, two days later the investigator showed up. She reviewed everything and promptly told me she was going to fine us $10,000 for this travesty. I just about had a heart attack in front of her. Instead, I followed Syp's instructions, maintained my composure, said nothing and let her leave in peace.

The next day Felipe returned. The Almond Joys grabbed me and asked to throw a welcome back party. I agreed and instructed the staff to help with whatever they needed. The party was a hit. There was music and refreshments all set up in the dining room filled with Ari's incredible handmade decorations. Dale used her excellent social skills and moved through the room with ease (or at least as far as a woman with a curved spine and walker could). When Felipe's wife and fourteen-year-old boy showed up, they joined in the festivities too. His wife was adamant that Liddy shouldn't be fired. She was sure it was an accident and Felipe really liked her. I promised her I'd do all that I could, but we had to wait until the state was finished with their investigation. I spent a little more time with her to see if they planned on suing us, and received only good feelings from her. As a result, I felt that I could turn my attention to other things and left the party early, thinking mostly about that $10,000 fine hanging over our head.

When I walked into my office, there, resting on my fax was a letter from Syp saying he'd taken care of the fine. It was now zero as evidenced by a letter from the state he sent too. Even better, the state had cleared Liddy of any wrongdoing. It was labeled 'Accident Due to Equipment Malfunction.' Relieved, I picked up the phone to call Liddy and give her the good news. "Liddy, you're in the clear. You can come back to work. Felipe and his family are asking for you."

Once I heard her response my good feelings turned sour. "Susan, thank you for the investigation and all the support, but I won't be coming back to the home. I've decided to take another job. During my time off I applied at a General Dollar store, and when the general manager reviewed my job application along with my last job evaluation, he hired me at the same salary I'd been making as a CNA. I want you to know this wasn't an easy decision, but I just can't come back after what happened. I know it was an accident, but the trauma of the whole thing is something I'll never forget. I just don't want to be responsible for someone getting hurt ever again, even if it wasn't my fault. I have to move on. I hope you understand."

I hung my head. "I understand. Really I do. You're going to be a great asset to the general manager and the company. We'll miss you terribly and so will Felipe. But I do thank you for your honesty and wish you all the best."

With that, I needed to start looking for another CNA.

It had been a month since the accident and everything was back to normal. During that time I'd been watching Ari and trying to learn more about him. Whenever I spoke to him, he talked in quotes relating to the question I asked. It was hard to get information that way. I watched his interactions with Dale. He followed her around like a puppy, almost looking to her for instructions on what to do. Dale, for her part, straightened his collar, wiped food off his shirt and made sure he was always taken care of. She was able to both understand what he was trying to say and translate for him. It was an opposite sex, dependent relationship without the sex; more like a very close brother-sister relationship. It was also obvious that Ari meant a lot to Dale's wellbeing. If one of them passed away, the other wouldn't be far behind.

I'd also been studying Ari's medical records. Wanting to know more about how the court got a hold of him and if it was legit, I called him into my office one day to see what I could find out. Predictably, Dale came with him.

"How are you two doing?"

"Smooth sailing ahead," said Ari.

"We're fine," Dale added.

"Good. Ari, I'd like to talk to you about your medical records. Would you like to do this privately or with Dale present?"

"The more the merrier," he replied.

"Okay, that's fine. What I really want to know is how you came to Warm Heart. How did you get under a guardianship? And if you're willing, I'd love to hear about your earlier life and bring it forward for me, so I can learn more about you."

We waited for him to begin speaking and when he did, he let out a string of quotes. Sometimes he added a sentence here or there that filled in the gaps, but it was hard for me to follow. That's when Dale began translating. After each translation, she asked him if it was correct and he gave some affirmative answer or quote. It was a bizarre way to communicate, yet somehow it worked. Here's what I learned:

Ari Stephenson was born in 1926. He had two sisters, both of whom were teenagers when they died tragically in an automobile accident. His parents were well educated and strict, but not abusive. He went to college, got a degree in engineering and worked for airline manufacturers like Lockheed-Martin and Boeing. He met his wife in high school, though they didn't date seriously until he was halfway through college. They lived slightly above middle class and never had any kids, although they'd talked about adopting. When they were both sixty-three, she died of cancer. He never got over it and never remarried.

He seemed to have a gift of fixing people when they were sad and lonely, sort of like a counselor without a degree. On the side, he yearned to go to Spain, though he never got to go there. Instead, he read all kinds of books about it.

The way he ended up in a nursing home was tragic. During his wife's illness, he was extremely dedicated to her wellbeing. When she fell ill, he went way beyond his limits to help her survive. By the time she died, Ari was completely depleted. He had not taken care of himself and the stress had taken a huge toll on his body. He was hospitalized for a raging infection a mere two days after his wife's funeral. He was treated and released with the understanding that he'd get regular checkups.

Yet Ari was not only depleted physically, he also was depleted financially. He'd spent every penny on his wife's healthcare and had almost nothing left over. Soon, his house was foreclosed on and the only shelter he had left was his car. Because he didn't eat right nor keep his blood pressure in check, he was soon hospitalized again. They diagnosed him with memory problems and that's when APS was called in. The same court that put Dale under a guardianship snagged Ari, too. His guardian treated Ari the same as Dale was treated—uncaring, unwilling to listen, and distant to his needs. When he met Dale, she became his blessing. Without her, he had no one to believe in him.

Now that he was in a nursing home, it was hard for Ari to believe and understand that he'd become weak and basically helpless. He had never thought age would catch up with him. And he was devastated that he'd run out of money before he ran out of life. It was a huge miscalculation.

When it came to Gracie, Ari loved her too, but he didn't like the cussing. He was always trying to give her 'better and nicer' words with his quotes. Sometimes Gracie would catch on, and sometimes not. But even the smallest changes in Gracie's vocabulary made Ari happy; it let him feel like he was helping to refine her vocabulary. He adored Gracie's daughter Mae and her grandchildren with all his heart. Even though Mae had some learning problems, she was the sweetest kid. She could make Ari feel so great about himself. It was like a holiday event every time Mae came to visit. I could see that girl was a blessing to both him and Dale, for they loved her so much. I could also see that Ari was both super smart and a very kind gentleman. He told me "the ear was the beginning and the end" and listening was the most important skill. The more I sat there, the more he reminded me of the actor Spencer Tracy. He just had that aura.

As far as my inquiry into the guardianship, it seemed legitimate. He had some mental problems, which they had recognized and then appointed someone to handle his affairs. After all, living in a car wasn't normal behavior for someone in their sixties. Still, he had detailed the same kind of poor treatment by his guardian as Dale and Ari did. It made me wonder.

We were about to wrap up it up when a man with a clipboard came in. "I just need a signature, ma'am."

"What's going on?" I asked, surprised.

"Delivery."

"Of what?"

"A Geri chair."

"A Geri Chair? How?!"

He stopped and looked at the clipboard. "Let's see, a Sen. K. B. Hutchinson. Do you know him?"

"Kay Bailey Hutchinson?! She's our senator, and I guess yours too."

He coughed. "Uh, I can't afford no senator. I'm just a delivery guy. Where do you want it?"

Before I could respond, Dale blurted out, "We'll show him!"

I jumped up and said, "No, we'll all show him."

We went to the lobby and watched eagerly as he lowered a ramp and wheeled in a brand new Geri chair covered in plastic wrap. It was a beautiful blue and shined brightly as we rolled it down the hall to Felipe's room. When we arrived, Dale went in and said, "Felipe, we have a present for you."

Felipe couldn't see the chair so Dale picked up one of the hand mirrors on his dresser and showed him the chair. Tears formed in his eyes and in the eyes of more than a few observers. I walked out of the room and let them have their little party. The truth was, I was completely blown away that they had pulled this off. And from a senator. Wow! These three were something else.

That evening, the CNAs used the Hoyer lift to carefully lower Felipe into the Geri chair. He was then rolled to his first ever dinner in the Jones-Simms facility. What an incredible experience it was. I could tell it was sensory overload for him, but he wouldn't change a thing. It was like he was soaking up everything he could in case it never happened again. That night when I went home, I had that fantastic warm feeling in my heart. I truly loved my job and didn't think it could get any better.

For the next week Felipe attended at least one meal a day. That's when the Almond Joys came to my office requesting something new. Dale took the lead on this one. "Susan, we would like to make changes to the meal service. We'd like to get rid of the plastic lunch trays and have real plates and cups. No more cartons of milk and juice either."

I raised my eyebrows. "I see. Is that the way they did it at Warm Heart?"

"No, of course not. Their meals were more like a prison service than a proper retirement home."

"Yeah," Gracie said. "We were fucking prisoners over there. And there was nothing to do. We all got medicated, sat up straight, and drooled. That happens here, too."

"Well, the staff doesn't like it any more than you do."

"Look, we need a culture change!" Gracie said. "We want the tables to look pretty. And we want to choose our own food, too."

"Okay, that's a lot to digest—no pun intended. I'm going to have to look at our budget and see what I can do. This might take some time so you'll have to be patient with me."

"Okay," Dale said. "We trust you. We really do."

Gracie added, "Yeah Administrator, you're good people. I know you won't treat us like prisoners unless you really have to."

Not to be left out, Ari said, "It's hard to knock a good man down."

After they left, I remembered the residents at Wellington Hills. They'd had real plates and glasses, along with real napkins. Their tables each had nice tablecloths. Could we afford anything close to that? I didn't know. Besides the money, there would be a lot of people to talk to. This would take some hard work, but deep down I knew they were right. It was something I had to try and give them.

My first stop would be to talk with the dietician. She came in for a few hours three times a week to review the diets of current residents and set up any new ones we'd gotten in. When she came in the next time, we had a long talk. "Susan, the main way in which large groups of people are cheaply fed is with the institutionalized method. That's what you have here. Specific types and quantities of food are placed on a serving tray and given to the resident. There's no sharing of the food and that helps prevent diseases from being passed around. Since you have no glasses, your cleanup up is quick and the trays are washed off fast. The military, prisons, and schools all use this method. It controls every bit of the process and keeps the costs down."

"I get what you're saying, but they deserve better. They want to eat family style, like when they lived in their homes. My goal is to get a big, old bowl of mashed potatoes, a big, old bowl of gravy and a large platter of meat, and sit it all right down in the middle of the table and let them pass it around. If they want more potatoes they can have more potatoes because it's right there in the middle of the table. Can't we have that?"

"Probably not, though a few states allow it. It's called 'liberalized dieting.' The residents help themselves to whatever they want and as much as they want. Your costs go up, but so does the satisfaction of the resident. And it's not just the costs of the food. More insulin and other medications will need to be administered because they'll be eating things that aren't good for them. Texas doesn't have a law against it, but I think they'll smack us down anyway."

"I don't care. That's exactly what I want to do and I don't care about the medication stuff either. I'm going to try it!"

"Okay, you can try it but first you need to get Dr. Lowery to sign off on it. That doctor's order will help us when the state comes a-knocking, and trust me, they'll come a-knocking."

Dr. Lowery turned out to be easy. He wrote a letter prescribing it for all of the residents and said, "It's about damn time. Everyone says a resident shouldn't eat this or that because they have high blood pressure or bad sugar. Well, yeah they do. And guess what? They're gonna die some day. We can give them a shot of insulin to help control it. So what if it means more work for the nurse? They'll die one week earlier, but at least they had satisfying meals every day of their life. What's that worth? Go for it, Susan. We'll deal with the consequences later."

With his letter in hand I sat down with the social workers, CNAs and food service staff. They were upset when they heard my grand plan. The complaints ranged from, "It's too dangerous" to "It'll be tons of work." There was also, "The food belongs in the kitchen!"

"No, it doesn't," I said, slapping my hand down on the table. "This is *their* home and *their* kitchen and *their* food. They want it on the table and guess what? It's gonna be on the table!"

Several grumbled and threatened to quit, yet I didn't care. With or without them, we were forging ahead.

To start this grand experiment, I selected a dinner on Monday evening. This gave us a lot of time to work between lunch and dinner. I knew it would be a huge surprise to all of the residents. The white tablecloths I purchased turned our cheap tables into nice, restaurant-quality settings. We set down maroon placemats and a gold charger on top to hold their ceramic plate. Next to each charger was a full set of nice (but not too expensive) silverware. A real glass stood like a watchtower guarding each place setting. I looked over everything one last time and gave the signal to call the residents in.

As they began trickling in, the first ones clapped their hands to their mouths in amazement. Some had tears in their eyes. When the Almond Joys saw it they each cried too. Felipe was wheeled in and was overcome with emotion. "It's like being in a nice restaurant," he whispered.

With everyone seated at their place, we went around and took cloth napkins and set them in each resident's lap. No longer would we have bibs attached to their necks like babies. Now, they'd be treated like real adults. If they made a mess, we'd clean it up. After all, everything could be washed.

I took a cloth napkin and asked Dale, "May I lay this in your lap?"

She looked up at me as tears rolled off her cheeks. "Now I feel respected."

I gently set the napkin in her lap and moved to the next resident. Most of them were too stunned to speak.

For the first time in a very long time, they could hold a real glass with not just water in it, but ice too. We also brought out all the condiments and anything else they might want. Instead of having everything hidden from the residents, they could see it all and make their choices. It was all about control. Some residents hated carrots and didn't want any. Before, we had simply slapped it on their tray and told them to eat the carrots. Now, they had full control. *They!* Not my staff. I had constantly heard the phrase, "for their own good." Now I replied, "It's what *they* say is good. Period!"

There were no more straws in cartons. No more plastic anywhere. "Oh, you want another pork chop Mr. Taylor? No problem, help yourself to one of these beauties. Another piece of pie, Mrs. Rials? Here it is, pick one out." With large bowls of food everywhere, the residents could finally smell the food. They could see the bacon resting on top of the green beans along with the shaved almonds. They could salivate as they dished out their food, enhancing both their desire to eat and their digestion. It was truly revolutionary. Sadly.

With this new dining style we effectively threw out their dining cards—the ones that said: Mr. Taylor's favorite fruit is cantaloupe and he doesn't like tuna fish. We'd been serving Mr. Taylor the same dishes all his life because that's what was on his card. We never thought to ask him if he was tired of cantaloupe or wanted to finally try tuna fish. Now Mr. Taylor could decide what he wanted at each meal and how much. If he wanted a change of pace, he could do it. If he liked to stay with the same routine, he could do that, too. The control was back in his hands, along with steaming bowls of fresh food.

As I watched them dive in and enjoy this, I remembered what Dale had said. She was right. It was a matter of dignity and respect. And not surprising, it made an immediate difference in their attitudes which then made the staff happy. This one change raised the overall mood in the home by leaps and bounds. That's how powerful 'liberalized dieting' is.

It didn't take long before the staff had the routine down. The family members who showed up to visit loved it, too. In fact, families started bringing centerpieces and adding decorations. It was just an awesome, awesome thing.

One of the staff members suggested putting on some music during the meals, so we brought in a stereo and offered music from various classical, soft jazz and lite rock stations. We also walked around serving coffee—as much as they wanted. So what it affected their health. We had nurses and CNAs to deal with it. Most of the residents knew well enough what to watch out for.

We were three weeks into this new meal service when sure enough, the state sent someone to survey us. Like clockwork, they freaked out. I was pretty sure the world as we knew it was coming to an end. They notified the state dietician who came to our home and claimed we were spreading infections around. It was terrible. She predicted the residents would soon be carried out in body bags once the first infection spread. The moment she left the premises I was on the phone with Syp. He made a call to the head lady over the dietary program for the state of Texas and according to Syp, she said, "To hell with it! I don't care! We want the families to eat there too, and the adults to eat like they do at home." She immediately overrode the lower level bureaucrats and that was that. We were now legitimate. In time, we would entertain other nursing home operators and state inspectors who'd heard about the revolution going on at the Jones-Simms Nursing Center. They all braved the Red Nine area to come have a look. Really, you'd have thought we invented space travel or something.

As each nursing home industry visitor left, they took this concept back to their part of the world and made their residents happy. So I guess when it came to the Almond Joys, it really was possible to change the world, even if you were locked up in some end-of-the-line nursing home against your will.

13

I could see the home was changing, due in no small part to the Almond Joys. They were everywhere, all the time, and involved in everything. One morning a resident fell and they were right there to keep her calm until the nurses arrived. "Don't worry, sweetie," Dale said, kneeling next to the fallen resident. "We all fall. The nurses will get you fixed up as good as new. They're almost here."

I just happened on this scene and watched the fear on the resident's face gently melt away with each soft word from Dale's lips. While Dale calmed her down, Gracie was wheeling around yelling for nurses and cursing in the language that only she seemed to use. But it worked. Two nurses came running fast and began tending to the woman immediately.

Falls cause injuries, sometimes serious ones. Luckily, this one wasn't bad. The resident had some dark bruising, but no broken bones and certainly nothing that required hospitalization. While the staff wheeled her back to her room to recuperate, one of the old-time LVNs whispered to me. "In my day, we just tied the residents to the beds with sheets. That way, they never fell out. We felt it was awesome because they didn't fall and didn't break a hip or something worse."

I glared at her. "No, no, and no. We don't tie up our children so they don't fall off the bicycle and we're not going to tie up our elderly.

A resident has a right to fall and not to be restrained. As much as I hate to see them fall, we can't restrict their life to avoid it. End of discussion!"

She got the message, though we did start focusing on why residents fall and where they were when the fall happened. This led us to start setting up fall programs based on a resident's fall pattern and prevent them from happening. It wasn't perfect, but every little bit helped.

With the excitement of the fallen resident out of the way, the Almond Joys had something else to focus on and it wasn't long before I once again heard the call of "Administrator! Administrator!"

Only Gracie addressed me like that. I turned around to see her rolling up towards me with Dale and Ari in her wake—they couldn't walk as fast as she rolled. "Yes Gracie, what can I do for you?"

"We want to start another club."

I gave them a huge smile; the fact that they seemed to start a new club every week made me happy. It showed they still had room for excitement. The first one they created was a bridge club. Once a week they held a bridge tournament and at least fifteen residents showed up. Since then, it had been a regular event with light music and coffee, teas and snacks served. It was comical to watch since there was less card playing and more talking. Human interaction was what they really craved. If a deck of cards was the excuse to get them together, so much the better. Cards were cheap.

I cleared my throat. "What club are you thinking about forming now?"

"An auction club."

"What's an auction club?"

"You know, you create house dollars and residents can earn or win them for a variety of things, like helping another resident for example. Or winning our weekly bridge tournaments. Or making nice rocks in the walking club."

The walking club was another one they'd formed. This club took the residents (whoever wanted to go) around the neighborhood for a brisk walk. They occurred after breakfast and before 10 a.m., the deadline for when the area awoke and began living up to its reputation. Typically a LVN or two led the group on different paths of a quarter mile while several CNAs pushed the ones in wheelchairs. Along the way, the residents would pick up interesting rocks and bring them back to the home where, as part of the club activities, they would clean and decorate them. Then they would give the rocks to their friends and loved ones to put in their gardens. Our patio had a nice collection of them already, which I had to admit made the barren landscape look a whole lot better.

"What kind of things do you want to auction away?"

"Things the residents make and donate or maybe special foods or privileges. You know, whatever we can come up with. What do you think?"

"Gracie, I think it's a wonderful idea. I'll get right on it and talk to Beth (our activities director)."

"Good. Let me know if I can help," she said as she rolled away, leaving me in charge of coming up with the details of her new idea.

That afternoon I had a meeting with Beth to start planning out the auction club. She had some extra money in her budget and agreed to start buying gifts to auction off. She created the funny money by making copies of monopoly dollars and telling the residents they could earn it by attending special events, doing something special for another person, and winning contests. She started passing it out at the many clubs that the Almond Joys had set up, including the paint club (where residents painted fabric and paper to decorate the home), the computer club (where residents learned about using computers) and the sports club (where residents watched sporting events on the TV). We held our first auction on Friday. Three items were up for bid. The first was a bag of jellybeans. It went to the Almond Joys, who pooled their money to buy it. The second item was a nice terrycloth robe that went to one of the female residents. The final item was one hour a day for one full week of controlling the TV's remote control. This turned out to be one of the most popular items auctioned off because people wanted to watch their special programs on the big screen TV.

Throughout the bidding, I could tell the residents were getting fired up and that their hearts were probably pumping more blood and beating faster than they had for a while. At times they stood up to yell out their bids, pointing this way and that when the numbers got close. Several times, if a resident didn't have enough money and was intent on winning the item, they desperately looked around for people to partner with. When each auction was over, the excitement lingered in the air and in the big smiles of the residents as they talked about what might've been and how they would prevail next time. I could see this was clearly a fantastic activity, one that got every resident fully engaged. Everyone, that is, except Mr. G. He was the one who'd objected the most about letting the Warm Heart residents stay. He was a quiet, brooding man, somewhat pudgy and never wore a smile. He had received a lot of cash, but never bid on anything. It was odd because he'd made every event, where before he'd never much cared to engage in any activities. I thought for sure this auction would bring him out of his shell, but I was wrong.

After the first auction, Gracie immediately went to Felipe's room to feed him some of the jellybeans they had won. Dale stayed behind with Ari and mingled with the residents. I stood back and watched her work. She was quite the social wonder. I could see why she had owned and operated a business. She was a community person, one that wanted to connect with everyone. Ari loved that quality in her, probably because that was how his wife had been.

Then there was Gracie, the quick-tongued, sometimes-vulgar grain of sand that caused a pearl to form. While she could be irritating and demanding at times, her motives were always selfless. That's why she got away with it. She was the perfect complement to Dale, who was more like a slick politician and Gracie the muscle. Ari provided both women the male authority figure for whatever they proposed. He gave them momentum by nodding his head and spouting quotes. Believe me, when they were standing in front of you demanding some change or new program, they were a powerful force—a determined three-against-one. If they chose to assert their force on you, you felt it.

By now the entire staff had completely fallen in love with these Almond Joys. It was like the staff and the Almond Joys had melted together. They were usually the main topic of conversation. People followed what they did and where they went. It was better than any reality show. Even though I was the administrator, they were indeed running the joint. I have to admit they were doing a great job—I could see the sparkle of life brought back to the residents' eyes. It was truly amazing!

One day Dale suggested to me that the nurses' chairs needed replacing. They were extremely warped with large holes in them. Several leaned to one side and most had their fabric torn and covered over with generous amounts of duct tape. "We can do better Susan. These nurses are the backbone of our healthcare system in here. Can't we find some money to replace these?"

A few weeks later, I had them replaced. When the new chairs were wheeled in, the Almond Joys used the occasion to have a ceremony. Music was played as each broken chair was retired and its replacement put into service. Photos were taken of the first person to sit in the chair, like they were some kind of royalty. It was yet another way to break up the daily routine and create something out of nothing.

Now that the nurses were excited with the new chairs, I expected their performance to increase. It did, for most of them. However, one afternoon we discovered a dosing error. The LVN gave the wrong medicine to a resident. She failed in administering the five rights of medicating: the right resident, the right drug, the right dosage, the right time and by the right route. I jumped in and, along with my DON, did an immediate investigation. We discovered she'd been pulling a triple shift. It was insane. Many of our nurses worked double shifts—they worked eight hours with us and eight more with another nursing home. With some of them, we were their second shift, instead of the first. Incredibly, this nurse was working *three* shifts and napping when she could. She told the other nurses she needed money for something that had come up. Now, her reckless decision had led to a dangerous dosing error.

We informed the family, who were understandably upset. We notified the state and they were sending out an investigator. Naturally. I called Dr. Lowery, who examined the resident and told us to observe her for seventy-two hours. While all this was happening, I got on the phone with Syp and told him about the accident. He gave me the correct protocol to follow and told me who would likely be coming out. When we were finished with all that, I switched to another subject. "Hey Syp, I have these three residents here and each one is on that $45 probate court guardianship program, yet they seem very competent to me. In fact, for one of them, if we could find the right family member, she could make it without court supervision."

"So?"

"So? I want to help them, maybe get a lawyer to investigate. You know, help get them out of the court program."

"Whoa, whoa, whoa! Don't you remember what I told you?"

"Sure. So?"

"So?! Listen up. The guardians in the program? They don't want you looking into this. The banks holding all that money? They don't want you looking into this. The judges who rely on votes from the public? This is their pet program, one they trot out to stay in office. They don't want you looking into this. Your company? They make money keeping butts in the beds, so they don't want you looking into this. Nobody wants you looking into this. *Nobody!*"

I paused for a moment. "What about the poor people trapped in this court-imposed prison?"

"What about them? Do you think Ari can live on his own?"

This took me by surprise. "How did you know his name?"

"I get paid to know everything. Can Ari live on his own?"

"Well . . . uh . . . no."

"Is he incompetent?"

"I don't think so, but he has trouble communicating. I believe, with the right person, he could live independently."

"Are you absolutely sure, Susan? One hundred percent? Would you bet your life on it?"

"No, not my life."

"Uh huh. Not *your* life, but you'd be okay putting *his* life at risk. Does he even have a relative who'd take him?"

"No. He has no one."

"So you'd set him up in an apartment he'd have to pay for out of his own pocket. Does he have any money or assets?"

"Well, no. He's on Medicaid, which I'm assuming you already know. But Gracie had both money and assets."

"Oh Gracie. Can she live in her own?"

"Well no, but with some assistance she could live at home. Unfortunately, though, there's no one to take care of her. But back to Dale. She's the saddest case of all of them. She's lost everything."

"Yeah, she did. So when you get it all back for her, can she still run her antique store?"

I was utterly stunned with his knowledge, but I guess I shouldn't have been. "Boy, you sure do know everything."

"What's your answer?"

"No, probably not. Still, that's no reason to steal it from her."

"Okay, she gets some money from a judgment and lives in a better home. Does Ari go with her?"

"Oh no, he'd die—literally."

"So meddling around in this is gonna get people killed. Right?"

"You know, I really hate talking to you about this guardianship prison. You just aren't looking at it from the right perspective."

"And you're gonna have some pills forced down your throat, get woozy and be deemed incompetent if you aren't careful. I told you, Texas law allows a probate judge to just snap his fingers and poof, you're bankrupt and in a nursing home located in the vibrant Red Nine area. Does that sound like a good outcome?"

"But . . ."

"No 'buts' about it. Spend your energy helping Dale, Ari, and Gracie live happy and full lives in your home. Trust me, if you rip them from this place, you'll watch helplessly as bad things happen. They're already institutionalized, whether they deserve it or not. Their assets have already been stolen, whether they deserved it or not. Nothing you're gonna do will ever change that. Now I have to run. Goodbye!" *Click.*

A few days later the state came out and wrote us up for the improper dosing incident. They fined us $1,500, which Syp made disappear. I implemented a policy of no triple shifts and suspended the guilty LVN for a week. She promptly quit and found another home so she could keep working her triple shifts. I told the LVNs I'd be monitoring their double shifts and total hours worked each week in any facility. If their hours climbed too high, I'd let them go. That seemed to solve the problem.

Periodically, I had to talk to each resident and make sure they didn't have any complaints or issues I needed to be aware of. Since we now had ninety-three residents, I divided this up to see four each day. This worked out so that I visited with each resident about once a month. Usually, a visit would include going over their file, verifying information on their loved ones, asking if anyone was harming them and other general questions. One day I was visiting with Felipe and asked him how he was doing. I wasn't prepared for his answer.

"I feel like I'm stuck."

Concerned I asked, "What are you stuck in? Do I need to get the lift in here?"

"No, a different kind of stuck. I'm stuck between living a quality life like all humans should and going to heaven. You know, I really intended to go to heaven, but now I'm just stuck in this middle world. My son was barely six when I tried to hang myself and now he's fifteen. He's had to watch me suffer all this time."

I moved closer to his bed. "But Felipe, don't you think you taught some things to your son? You've been able to have a relationship with him."

"Yeah, sure. That's a good thing and so was Warm Heart closing down and bringing me the Almond Joys. They've truly been a godsend. But I know that I'm a burden to society and that's why I'm stuck. I need to get unstuck, especially since my ten years is about up."

"What ten years?"

"The doctors said I'd live like this for about ten years. That's the statistic. My son just turned fifteen, so I'm almost there."

Growing concerned, I said, "Let's not talk like that. You'll be with us for a long time, maybe even to see him married and have some grandchildren."

"No, I don't think so. I think it's time for me to go. To get unstuck."

"What can I do for you?"

"Pray."

I forced a smile. "Felipe, I do that every day."

"Thanks, Susan. I believe you."

I left his room and made a note to have the doctor talk to him. It sounded like he may need some psychological help. No sooner had I left and the Almonds Joys were wheeling in the projector to tell another story on his ceiling. They loved to entertain him before dinner because they wanted to watch the lift as it hoisted him from the bed and into his Geri chair. Then they'd walk with him to dinner. They stayed attached to him like his life depended on it, and perhaps it did.

The next morning I drove up to work and saw flashing lights. A gurney was leaving an ambulance that was parked in front of our home. In a rush, I forgot to pray as I entered my side door and hurried to the nurses' station to find out what had happened.

"It's Felipe," Cayla said. "He's dead."

"What?!" I covered my gaping mouth with trembling hands.

"Yes, we found him when we went to get him for breakfast. The CNA was confused because his eyes were open and he had a smile on his face."

"Are you serious?" I couldn't believe what I was hearing.

"Yes, I saw it myself."

I went down to Felipe's room and saw the sheet over him as they loaded his body onto a gurney. There the Almond Joys were, tears streaming down their faces. Usually they consoled others, but now it seemed the entire home was there hugging Dale, Gracie and Ari. As the gurney rolled past them, precisely three jellybeans fell from the folds of Felipe's clothes. The three picked them up, each one absolutely sure it was sign from Felipe telling them that he was going to be all right. I have to admit, it hard not to become emotional seeing all this. They loved him so very much.

When Felipe's family came to the home, the Almond Joys hugged them like long, lost family. I was amazed how close total strangers could become. Two weeks later I learned his autopsy showed he'd died of a brain aneurism. Just like he'd hoped for, Felipe had finally become unstuck.

Beth, our activities director, had been working with Gracie and Dale to bring in more outside talent for events. One person they'd liked at Warm Heart was a singer named Blue-zy. One evening, we set up an event after dinner where she came and entertained the home by singing to prerecorded music. It was a fine show by a talented singer, one I stayed late to watch. After the show, I had fun talking with Blue-zy and learned that she'd lived an exciting life, traveling throughout the world and playing in large venues. She was retired now, but still loved singing and working out her vocal cords. These days, though, she performed in venues like this. I made sure that she knew we were blessed to have her.

We passed out Deed Dollars, as we called them, to all who came to the event. The next day—Friday—we held another auction. I was eager to see how this one would go. In the past several months, pretty much every resident had bid on and won something. Today, we were auctioning off the usual assortment of stuff, but we also included a perfectly round, ripe watermelon—the kind with bright green and dark green strips around it. Since this was July, the fruit was at its sweetest.

I was particularly curious to see if this would entice Mr. G (or 'Mr. Grumpy') to bid. He still hadn't bid on anything. We figured he was sitting on quite an impressive stack of Deed Dollars. The first items went without him batting an eyelash. Then it was time for the watermelon. The bidding was frenzied—we rarely had watermelon to serve to our residents. Twelve bidders pushed the price up to $1,000 in just five minutes. That's when two dropped out due to lack of funds. Then the amount rose again and three more quit. Then two more were gone. Now, five were left and none of them were Mr. G. When the price rose to $2,500, only two had that amount, but barely. One of them outbid the other to $2,501. Before the other bidder could counter, Mr. G, for the first time ever, stood up and yelled with as much gusto as he could. "$3,000!" The two bidders looked at each other, sank down into their chairs and threw up their arms. The game was over.

"C'mon on up and get your watermelon, Mr. G." He shuffled up and carefully counted out his money, which appeared to be all he had. As he returned to his seat, he cradled that melon like it was a newborn child. In fact, he walked the halls holding that watermelon for the next two days. None of us were sure if he was showing it off or trying to decide what to do with it. When the sports bar club was trotted out for a baseball game, he brought his melon to a table where he could watch the game. That's when he asked for a knife. Carefully slicing it down the middle, and then into smaller pieces, he spent the next hour devouring every square inch of the juicy, red flesh. By the time he was done, red juice had dripped from his face all over his clothes, which were a big mess now. Like a conquering general leaving behind the carnage on the battlefield, Mr. G rose from the table and quickly made his way to the restroom—the massive water content stored in watermelons had apparently reached his bladder.

Through the red mess on his face, I definitely saw a smile wrinkling his cheeks—the first one I could ever remember.

That day, many of the residents were overjoyed to see Mr. G happy. He never bothered anyone, and besides looking perpetually grumpy, seemed in need of a hug. The Almond Joys were constantly trying to bring him out of his shell. We figured it had been hardened from years of living in a nursing home on Medicaid. He had no other money nor any visitors or relatives to share a moment with. It was sad.

When the festivities came to an end, I went back to my office and closed the door, smiling at the newfound memory of Mr. G and his watermelon. Relaxing back in my chair, I glanced over at to the fax machine and saw a fresh fax lying there. It was from the state of Texas. It read, "After a review of your facility's records for the past six years, you owe $3,051,754.23. Please remit payment within ten days." I dropped the fax and almost fainted.

14

"Here we go again," was the phrase racing through my mind. Over three million owed. I couldn't believe what I was seeing. It was insane. While I sat there trying to get my heart rate back to normal (or as close to normal as possible), I studied the fax carefully. Apparently they'd done an audit for the past six years—five of which I wasn't here—and decided our billings had been miscoded. Or an 'i' wasn't dotted. Or perhaps there had been a smudge on a piece of paper. Whatever their reasons, we just needed to come up with three million in cash and everything would be fine. Actually, it was our mother company that was on the hook since they inherited these problems when they had purchased the place. That still didn't make me feel any better.

After a few minutes of panicking, I picked up the phone and called Billy. I figured he was the first who needed to know. Unfortunately, he was in a high level meeting and unavailable so I left a message for him to call me. Then I dialed Syp.

"Yeah," he answered bluntly.

"It's me, Susan. I have a problem."

"You mean you have a $3,000,000 problem."

Once again I was stunned. "You already know about it?"

"Yeah, they hit all of our homes and just about every facility in Texas. I think it's a budget deal. They're out of money and shaking down the industry, seeing how much they can dig up."

"So you know the exact amount?"

"Sure," he said, almost bored. "They sent a certified letter to your corporate office days ago, along with the other homes, too."

Suddenly, I felt better. "Okay, is there anything I can do?"

"Nothing at this point. We may need some records, but just go back to running your facility and be ready for some transfers. Some of the smaller mom and pop homes will have to close. They can't afford to fight it or hire a guy like me."

"All right. Thanks for letting me know. You always seem to calm me down during these hectic times. I'm glad you're on our team."

I hung up and called Melva into my office, recapping the whole affair.

"That's crazy," she said. "At my last job we were audited and had $60,000 in disputed charges. I thought that was bad, but this is almost comical."

"I know, but I'm not laughing. I about had a heart attack when I read it."

"No doubt. I probably would've too. But on a positive note, I just got off the phone with the probate court lady, Nala Stahl. When Mrs. Blandon died, I didn't send in her $45 court fee. I figured she didn't need any more supervision once she was dead. Nala, on the other hand, explained that she was still living during three out of the four weeks of that month. Therefore, we needed to send in the money. Since they didn't have a death certificate from us, they were still providing services. She was hotter than a firecracker!"

"I thought you said 'on a positive note'?"

"I did," she said chuckling. "The positive note was when I got off the phone."

I frowned. "Great, so now the burden is on us to show them a person they're supposed to be supervising is dead. How rude of us."

Melva tapped my desk with her finger. "Yeah, she was pretty threatening, too—the judge can do this and the judge can do that. You know, blah, blah, blah. Man they think they have a lot of power over there."

I took a deep breath. "According to Syp, they do. Even he seems scared of them. He's told me over and over to leave them alone."

"Well, don't worry, I'll deal with her. If I turn up missing, start there."

"I will. But honestly, that's not funny."

"Wow, you sure are a grouch today," she said sarcastically. "I guess nothing's funny after you get a $3,000,000 notice."

She was right. This was becoming a very bad day.

I left the office late and walked to my car, spotting our trash dumpster at the far end of the parking lot. Next to it was a recycling bin. I squinted my eyes and saw two people rummaging through everything. Or actually one person rummaging while another person sat in a makeshift wheelchair that looked to be part secretarial chair and part grocery cart. They were oblivious to my presence so I stood there for a few minutes, watching.

I could tell they were looking for pieces of equipment we'd dumped, as they obviously needed some spare parts to make handicapped equipment for themselves. The first time I'd seen something like this was six months earlier when we'd placed a broken bedside table on the curb. Soon after, a homeless person had spent hours removing one wheel for his rolling chair. The next homeless person came along and removed yet another wheel for something. Two days later the entire table had been devoured, leaving nothing for the trash haulers. I learned that they took just what they needed and left the rest for the next person. If the item could be fixed, they'd fix it and use it for something, or perhaps sell it. It was a strange and sad sight. This is what life looks like when you're poor and at the very bottom—picking through human fluids, spoiled food, waste-filled diapers, urine bottles, and whatever other nasty things are in there to find a piece of something to help you survive. I continually thanked God that wasn't me.

The next morning, after an uneasy night of sleep, I stopped at the door and said my usual prayer. This time I added a bit about getting us out from under the $3,000,000 debt. I thought it was only appropriate since we'd probably need a miracle.

As I made my usual rounds, I noticed the three Almond Joys bouncing around happy and joyous to be alive. They had been essentially kidnapped and financially raped, yet here they were, unwilling to waste their final years wallowing in misery. And here I was, trying to smile but dying inside. I wanted them to know how terrible I felt, but the news I held would likely scare them. So while they did their thing, I suffered in silence.

I approached Ari and said, "Good morning."

He looked at me with a sparkle. "Always try to become a person of value—Albert Einstein."

"That's right. I always try to be that. Thank you Ari."

I was standing in the activity area where Dale and Gracie had butcher block paper spread on every table. The residents were dabbing on little sponges of color and other decorative stamps. Dale had sharpies and was helping each participant write inspiring comments and sign their names on the paper. Beth, our activities director, also had several brushes for the acrylics. It looked like everyone was having a good time. Then I saw Mr. G. His hands were deep in paint, having put aside the brushes for a more direct approach. Gracie was next to him, urging him on while throwing in a few pointers. He'd been like a different person ever since the watermelon auction. Now, he engaged with people and had become one of the most liked residents. It was as though we had a whole new person in the home.

When one of the artists finished their creation, they went through the home trying to decide where to hang it. A few ended up in the residents' rooms, but most decorated the halls and common areas for everyone to enjoy and comment on.

From my first day on the job, one thing Billy was adamant about was urging a new resident to bring something from their home to their new room. It could be a recliner, coffee table, trinket, or something special that would not only remind them of home, but also help them adjust to their new place. The Almond Joys had learned about this policy and took it a step further. When a resident had a visitor, they urged them to bring something from home for our dinner table, some decoration they might have lying around. This could be something personal they put together or something they had purchased. Several visitors even searched through their attics, finding old centerpieces and bringing them in for the Almond Joys to clean up and make new. Now, each meal had rotating centerpieces, most of which held a personal meaning for one of the residents. It was a brilliant idea that made the meals even that much more special.

Besides working in the common areas, the Almond Joys were knee deep into fixing up each resident's room, or at least the ones who wanted them fixed up. Each Monday they'd pick a room and start decorating. It could be something simple, like washing the old curtains or getting some new fabric and making new ones. They might specifically design butcher-block paper posters for a room. One resident was a huge Dallas Cowboys fan, so they decorated the paper with blue and silver. Another piece of paper listed the Cowboys' upcoming schedule with a place to write down the final scores. When they were done, his half of the room looked like it belonged in the Dallas Cowboys' locker room. Because his neighbor liked forest scenes, they taped fake plants to the walls and painted butcher paper to look like trees. They even painted glow-in-the-dark stars on the ceiling (or had one of the CNAs do it). If you turned the lights out it actually felt a little like a forest.

They also made sure every resident had plenty of photos of relatives on the walls. If they didn't have money for frames, they made some out of cardboard and decorated them. Some of the cardboard frames had a wood grain pattern. Nothing was out of reach for these three characters. Never in a million years could I have foreseen three people having such a huge impact on the lives of so many people. Ninety-plus residents, their relatives, a hundred employees and of course, me. They were truly a blessing.

A clap of thunder brought me back to reality. I jogged to a window and saw a strong storm in progress. A solid wall of rain pounded the pavement outside and large pools of water rapidly formed. I heard shouts behind me and saw Carlos carrying several squeegees and push brooms. Right behind him were the Almond Joys. They carried as many towels as they could, with Ari the most heavily loaded down. By now they'd been through several floods and knew the drill.

In minutes the water was rushing into several parts of the building. Like always, Carlos and several CNAs fought to contain it to a general area. The Almond Joys continued to bring him supplies while making sure all the windows were closed in the residents' room. The Almond Joys' rooms were not in the flood-prone areas, so they could've easily sat back and watched the calamity. Instead, they knew it was their home and thus, their responsibility. Besides, I think they actually enjoyed emergencies such as these. It got their juices flowing and made them feel even more alive.

I was working side by side with our staff with a push broom in my hand when Mr. G came up and dropped several paper boats into the large lake on our floor. We all laughed. It was obvious that Dale or Gracie had planned ahead and assigned Mr. G this chore. The boats not only floated, but seemed to be on a journey to an unknown destination, drifting here and there as we pushed the water to a general holding area near the lobby. Each time we pushed the water, we created waves that sent the boats onward, enjoying their freedom on Lake Red Nine until the storm abated. It always seemed the more violent the storm, the quicker it passed and this one passed in ten minutes.

Though the water stopped coming in, the mess remained. Wet towels were everywhere. They were too heavy for most residents to lift, so the Almond Joys pushed them into a pile as best they could until Carlos came by with a wheelbarrow, loaded them up, and took them outside to ring out. Within an hour of the first water coming in, the floors were dry, the sun was out, and life was back to normal. Of course, the Almond Joys weren't superhuman. Even they required daily naps and with the energy they'd just expended, it was time for some big ones. When they went to sleep, it was like the pilot turning out the lights on a plane at night—everyone took a nap.

"Administrator, Administrator!"

Smiling, I turned around and said, "Yes Gracie, what can I do for you?"

"We need to arrange some date time." This was code for sex. Recently, a lady and a gentleman had gotten somewhat familiar with each other. The woman, wanting to have sex with her man, had been unwilling to approach any of the staff about it. So she went to Gracie, who was more than willing to be the middleman.

"I see. And who is it?" I knew who it was, but felt I shouldn't assume.

"It's Sheryl and Carson. You know, the usual."

Ms. Unger and Mr. Reindl. This was their third date and by now they were old hands at it. I'd made sure long ago that all my staff knew my policy on sex—a resident has a right to sexual activity. It happened to be the state's policy as well. They don't lose their lives just because they come into a facility. As a result we'd set up an arranged time and make sure they had the necessary tools: lubricant, pills, and privacy—the usual. It was our job to set them up for success.

Because the dates were usually in Ms. Unger's room, we arranged an activity for her roommate, Mrs. D'Angelo. She loved to play dominos, so it was easy to make happen. Gracie, Dale and Ari would pick up Mrs. D'Angelo at the appointed time and escort her to the activity area, where they would play dominos for an hour or so. Meanwhile, Mr. Reindl would saunter on in and close the door for a little Jones-Simms intimacy. I made sure my staff stayed away. After all, this was their home. We were just guests in it.

As fall approached and the football season started up, the Almond Joys asked to move the sports bar outside. The weather was nice which allowed us to roll out the big screen TV to the patio along with a stand-up bar. Dale had an idea to create a potato bar outside, so one Sunday before the game the staff cooked up a bunch of baked potatoes and took them outside with all the fixin's. Each resident took their potato and poured whatever they wanted on it. Mr. G was the most interesting to watch, as he meticulously piled every ingredient onto a separate part of the potato, not realizing he could simply place it on the surrounding plate. We all watched him set the potato down and carefully study it like it was a diamond he was about to cut. Finally, he dove in and like the watermelon, devoured every square inch.

At the end of September the Almond Joys suggested turning the sports bar into a real bar. I agreed and bought wine and beer, all non-alcoholic. The staff set up the bar one Sunday, placing newspapers out for them read, along with select dishes of pickled eggs, peanuts, pig's feet and other snacks. All the bottles of the non-alcoholic beverages were glass and shoved into ice buckets to properly complete the scene. This was one Sunday when I showed up because I personally wanted to serve them the 'alcohol.' I insisted on putting their drinks into red Solo cups in case they dropped them. The last thing I wanted was glass shattered everywhere. The residents were okay with this. It made them feel like they were at a real tailgate party.

To my surprise, though, some residents appeared to get tipsy. I checked the bottles to make sure there wasn't any alcohol in them. There wasn't. Still, as one of the female residents got a little goofy, another resident followed suit. Soon, at least ten of them were tipsy. As the game roared on, many of residents didn't care, and instead danced with one another to some music we had playing. An hour into this affair, they all looked like eighteen- or nineteen-year-olds throwing a party before their parents came home. It was absolutely amazing! Their depression and health ailments seemed to dissipate into thin air as the fake drinks went down. They were happy, even Mr. G. And all because the drinks looked and tasted like alcohol.

After it was over, Dale and Ari picked up cigarettes butts while Gracie loaded up supplies on her wheelchair to carry inside. They were the hosts of the party and now that it was over, they felt a duty to clean up.

A few days later, Mr. G developed a bad cough. The doctor prescribed some medicine for him, but it didn't help. The Almond Joys tended to him religiously, just like they'd done for Felipe. One night, Gracie was in there talking to him when he had trouble breathing. Because she knew something wasn't right, she wheeled out into the hall and yelled, "Nurse! Nurse!"

They came running and tried desperately to help Mr. G, but he passed away before we could even call 9-1-1. He died right in front of them. It was a tough blow, not only for the residents but for the staff, too. We had all really grown to love this tough teddy bear.

Ari went into the room just as they lifted the sheet over his face and said, "Let it be done."

Because Mr. G had been on Medicaid for many years, he had no money for a funeral or a burial plot. He was to be buried in a public cemetery with no marker. This didn't sit well with the residents. They held a meeting, which resulted in the Almond Joys visiting my office.

"Administrator, we want you to call the public cemetery and see if we can assist in the burial. We've talked with several of the staff and they've volunteered to dig the hole."

"Gracie, are you kidding me?"

"No, we're not." It was Dale speaking up. "If we pay to have a hole dug for him, can we pick out his gravesite?"

I shook my head. "I need to tell you this is extraordinary, but I'll call them to find out if any of this is even possible."

Dale wasn't finished. "Also, if we can pay for a marker, could you find out how much that would be?"

I held up a hand. "Listen, I'm going to try to find out what we can do, but don't get your hopes up. The public cemetery is run by a government agency and you know how government agencies are."

"We understand," Dale said. "But please do your best. Please. Mr. G meant a lot to all of us."

"Yeah, Administrator. Do what you can."

I nodded my head as they stood to leave. Ari waited behind and made one last comment, "He was a good man and the world needs more good men."

"Agreed."

I set to my task with all the determination I could muster. After reaching the proper governmental agency, I discovered that we could not assist with digging the hole. No surprise there. The man practically laughed into the phone. As for the marker, he said we'd have to cough up $2,000. No one had that kind of money, at least not that they could afford to turn loose. The residents were crestfallen when I gave them the news.

A week later I took a trip to the cemetery and learned where Mr. G was buried. I went to my car and took out an old blanket, one I'd sewn burlap backing to. Then I dumped a dozen packages of wildflower seeds into the burlap sack and took it to the gravesite. Laying the blanket over Mr. G's resting place, I took six one-gallon water jugs and dumped them over the blanket, soaking the seeds while creating some mud on the dirt around the edges. I got down on my hands and knees and smoothed an inch of mud over the burlap sack and packed it hard. To complete the operation I walked all over it forcing it to sink down even farther, hopefully obscuring it from the groundskeepers who'd surely pick it up and throw it in the trash. When I was done, I went to my car and laid another blanket over my seat, trying my best to keep my car clean.

For the entire next week, I dropped each day to pour more water over his grave. I didn't know if what I was doing was illegal or could impact my license, but I didn't care. About three weeks later, I saw a wonderful sign: sprouts bursting through the mud with the first flower opening up. Now it was time to share all this hard work by arranging a field trip for the residents. But first, I had to get them here.

We had a rickety old bus that belonged to our home. I laid some sweet talk on Billy and convinced him to provide two more buses with drivers. We loaded everyone onboard who wanted to come and took off. After we arrived, we gathered around Mr. G's gravesite where they all proceeded to cry. There, on his 3 x 8 rectangle, were densely packed wildflowers. One of the residents said, "God has taken care of Mr. G by personally making a marker for him. God must've really loved Mr. G to do that for him."

I nodded my head in agreement. I knew God had given me this plan and I had only carried out His wishes.

Gracie rolled up to within an inch of the grave and said this prayer, "Dear Lord, with Mr. G you got a damn good soul!"

Ari, Dale and other residents responded, "Amen."

It was a wonderful day indeed.

When we got back and unloaded everyone, there was a fax waiting on my desk. It said the state of Texas was reducing our $3,000,000 fine to $9,576. I laughed, because I knew either Syp or God had something to do with it and right now, I was betting on God. That's why I wasn't surprised when, with the empty bed Mr. G left behind, a new person showed up the next day to take his place. That person was Bulldozer.

15

I first heard about Bulldozer when a doctor's office called, looking to place him in a nursing home. Billy had relationships with many of the doctors in the area which meant they usually called us first when they had a patient with no money who needed a facility like ours. In this case, Melva talked to the doctor, got all the details, and plugged the data into the state's computer. After it spat out a high RUG rate, we were happy to accept him, as he would need a lot of services.

"When is he coming?" I asked Melva.

"Today. He's been tying up a hospital bed for four weeks. When the ambulance arrives, a hospital nurse will be here to help move him in. She's going to stay with us for half a day to make sure our staff understands everything he needs—the IVs, drugs, dressings, etc. The doctor told me they'd make sure he was comfortable because he won't be leaving this facility after he's situated. His name is Stewart Compton and he's a lifer."

"How old did you say he is?"

"Thirty-four."

"Oh my! That's way too young. What happened?"

Melva picked up her notes papers. "According to the medical records, he worked in construction. One Friday, he was paid $500 in cash instead of given a check. There was a girl he was interested in so he asked her out on a date. She agreed and told him where she lived. The problem was, she didn't really live there. It was an abandoned home, one of those old ones with big steps leading up to a wide porch. There were bushes on either side and when Stewart went to pick her up, some man jumped out from a bush and shot him three times. They took his cash and left him for dead. Neighbors heard the gunshots and found Stewart lying there. The hospital saved his life, but said he was essentially paralyzed due to severe muscle and bone damage."

I whistled. "Wow! That's a tragic story. Did they catch the people who did this?"

"You bet. Both the girl and the shooter have been arrested and are facing decades in jail. The doctor told me the police would probably want our medical records for the trial."

"Okay, they'll be in order and hopefully these people can spend the rest of their lives in prison. Let's get ready to receive him. Do you have a room picked out?"

Melva smiled. "Yes, Mr. G's old spot. It gets the morning sun and might make him feel better when he wakes up. Besides, it's two doors down from Gracie. That ought to work out very nicely." I grinned because I knew exactly what she meant.

The delivery and installation of Stewart went smoothly. Once he was in his bed, Gracie rolled down to greet him. Within an hour after that, the place was buzzing about the Almond Joys new project— Bulldozer. By the time the hospital nurse left, the Almond Joys knew his entire life story and complete medical history. When I walked in to meet him, they were already feeding him a few jellybeans and putting a production on his ceiling. He seemed dazed by all of the attention.

I introduced myself and let him know I'd be around later to go over his rights and collect the names of any visitors he might have in the future. Then I left him in the capable hands of our nurses and, of course, the Almond Joys.

Over the next few weeks his demeanor went from one of acceptance to one of determination. At the Almond Joys' urging, he decided he'd walk again and eventually get out of the home. They promised to help. In fact, they set up posters to track his progress. Each day he saw what he'd done the day before and tried to exceed it. It was always staring him right in the face.

His first goals were simply to lift his arms and legs half an inch off of the mattress. It took a week, but he managed to do it. It was much more than the doctors ever thought he'd achieve. I watched him do this exercise once and saw how hard he had to work just get one arm or leg off the bed. I knew right then that he'd never leave our facility, but I didn't want to rain on the Almond Joys' parade. Besides, God had worked a miracle on the $3,000,000, so I knew He could help Bulldozer.

By the end of the first month, everyone was pulling for him. He was by far the youngest resident we'd ever had, so we all knew he didn't truly belong here. And his sweet, likable personality also made it easy to root for him.

The Almond Joys weren't satisfied to help just one person. They wanted more. They got with Beth and set up a reading club. Due to poverty or nationality, several of our employees had a hard time reading. The Almond Joys also knew this. They began working with a few people during their breaks and soon showed real progress. Within a couple of weeks the employees started bringing in their children to have them join the reading club. Dale would stand up and tell stories, capturing the little ones' attention. At the same time, Gracie and several other residents would pull out books and read next to the student. Ari mainly hovered around, getting books and waiting on people. This reading club was yet another wonderful project started by these three people.

Once the reading club was going well, they met with me again to set up a country store. The idea was to sell items to the residents directly, rather than having someone go out and get it piecemeal. In other words—buy in larger quantities. They wanted to sell soaps, special snacks, greeting cards and dozens of other items that we knew the residents often purchased. The profit from the country store would go to fund the various clubs, in particular the reading club. The Almond Joys wanted more books and reading tools. I agreed, so long as the residents ran the store themselves and kept the financial records. We couldn't afford to pay for all of the country store's expenses. Fortunately, one of the residents—Mr. Reindl—used to be an accountant and he agreed to handle the bookkeeping. It seemed to energize him, much like his occasional rendezvous with Ms. Unger. Eventually the store was up and running an hour each day with Mr. Reindl handling everything, including making sure all of the products were locked up once it closed. The profit from the country store easily funded the other clubs. It was great!

Three months into the country store project, clothing was added. This came about when it was time to change out the residents' wardrobe to get ready for winter. Twice a year we went to a warehouse behind the facility and took out the residents' stored clothes. The warm things they kept for winter were switched out with the summer attire they'd been wearing for months. This was not only an exciting deal, but also an important one. Elderly people experience temperature changes more keenly, and in the winter they're prone to feeling cold all the time. They really love it when it's hot. For summer, we dress them in thin shirts and shorts to allow the heat to soak into their bodies. But in the winter they need thick, warm clothing. Since their closets are about two feet wide, they couldn't have all of their clothes readily available. That's why the stored clothes came out at the change of the seasons. Unsurprisingly, many of the residents found one or two items that didn't fit or look as good as they remembered. It just so happened that one of our employees worked at Target as a second job and had access to all the stuff that didn't sell. We'd buy the clothes at a huge discount and sell them to the residents for a profit. This store really allowed them to feel in control of some aspect of their lives and made them happy.

I noticed Dale was one of the first to buy clothes. She was beginning to hunch over more and more and was wearing out a few dresses as they dragged around on the floor. She was also losing just a bit of energy. Still, she outworked and out-greeted anyone else in the home (although Gracie gave her a good run for her money). Dale was the captain that steered the Almond Joys' ship.

They had been in our home for a year when I realized how much the state survey results correlated to their presence. As a nursing facility administrator, a survey is like a report card for how well I'm doing my job. It tells me what I need to do to improve operations and points out any violations. Sometimes they even issue a fine. Ever since the Almond Joys had joined the home, the state surveys were all outstanding. I was under no allusions as to how that had happened. I just hoped they would live as long as my career lasted.

One day I received a call from my good friend Vicki. "Susan, I need to talk to you!" She sounded panicked.

"What is it? Are you okay?"

"I hope so," she said out of breath. "The lady from the probate court, Nala Stahl, was here auditing our books. We were missing the records of one resident and hadn't paid a few months of fees on another—completely by accident. Now she's threatening to pull both residents from our home. She was very aggressive. It sounded like I'd be hauled before the judge and required to answer for my crimes. Has this happened to you?"

"No, it hasn't. Melva deals with her, thank God. We did have a problem over something, but I can't remember the details. You really sound scared."

"Yeah, it kinda has me frazzled. It's like these residents belong to the probate court and they're furniture that can be repossessed and moved around wherever they want. It just so happens several of her units—if I can call them that—have high RUG rates. Right now we're just above our minimum capacity for making a profit and I can't afford to lose them. I don't think she knows this, but who knows?"

"I understand. A consultant who works for our company seems scared of her too, and he's been able to get everything done. It's bizarre. We're up to twelve under the court's program and maybe half of them look like they could live on their own. They don't seem incompetent, or at least, not to me. Heck, I can't remember what day it is half the time. I think if they tested me I'd end up in their prison."

"Yeah, and broke, too. They suck up their assets like a vacuum cleaner. Someone has to be getting rich on all this."

The more we talked, the more she calmed down. We were trained to deal with health inspectors, state investigators, local protective service agencies and even the media. But nowhere had we ever learned about dealing with judges who could simply drop the gavel and have someone committed against their will. It seemed like something dictators in third world countries did, not a free country like America. When Vicki and I were finished, I called Melva in and made sure we were in good standing with the probate courts. She assured me we were. Since Vicki's problem wasn't affecting me personally, I quickly put it out of my mind and worried about other things. That was a big mistake, one that would eventually cost lives.

With all the clubs the Almond Joys had set up, I finally realized that the key to keeping the residents from getting depressed—to help them look forward to getting up in the morning—was to give them jobs and responsibilities. Mr. Reindl was a good example. He ran the country store and it gave him purpose. Two of the residents who worked in the reading club now felt like the world needed them. They made it their personal goal to get someone reading. Getting and keeping them interested in something was the key.

One event everyone in the home was greatly interested in was the presidential election. Everywhere there were banners and signs supporting both candidates. Each resident was encouraged to vote and given access to the polls. On Election Day we had the televisions tuned in for wall-to-wall coverage. Once the polls closed, everyone huddled around the big screen TV watching the vote totals as each state came in. When they projected a winner, many of the viewers cheered. Since a lot of the staff and residents were African-American, they were both speechless and overwhelmed when Barak Obama won. Several cried. The next morning, the Almond Joys started talking about having a Jones-Simms inauguration. I liked the idea. Beth knew a person who rented party dresses and tuxedos and she let us use her wardrobe for free. She brought boxes of clothing to the home for the residents to pick out something nice to wear. Of course, the staff helped them with all this too.

On the big day, the food staff concocted a special meal for dinner, something roughly similar to the food they were serving at the real inauguration: seafood stew, pheasant with sour cherry chutney (we used chicken), wild rice stuffing, sweet potatoes, winter vegetables, and apple-cinnamon sponge cake. The Almond Joys worked hard to make elaborate presidential centerpieces and other decorations, which they hung around the dining area. For Bulldozer, they dusted off Felipe's old Geri chair and supervised the CNAs as they gently lifted him into it. Like Felipe, they made sure he was included in every event.

Another staff member knew a DJ who, without charge, came and put on music like a regular party. I bought more nonalcoholic beverages and served them all night long, watching again as many of the residents became 'tipsy.' After dinner, all the residents who could dance did. By the time the affair was over, the residents were both exhilarated and thoroughly exhausted. It was yet another great experience.

A week after the inauguration, Bulldozer went back into the hospital to have another surgery. When he fully recovered, he had more flexibility. This is where the CNAs used what little rehab equipment we had to try to get him moving more. And the Almond Joys were there, urging him on every step of the way. It was truly amazing when, one month later, he was walking between the bars on his own. It did, however, take at least ten minutes and a lot of arm work. Still, I thought about that miracle again.

Just as things were going great, something always popped up and knocked me back to reality. One day a nurse locked up her purse in the medicine storage area and went back to tending to residents. Minutes later, a check cashing place called me to make sure the nurse whose name was on the check worked at our facility.

"Yes, she does," I said confused. "When does she want to cash it?"

"Right now. She's standing in front of me."

"What?! That's impossible. I'm looking at her right now through my office door. How can she be there and here at the same time? Wait a second."

I called the nurse over and told her what was going on. She ran to check her purse and found the check was missing. "Let's drive down there," she said. "It's only three blocks away."

I told the check cashing man to keep the person there so we could come and identify her. He said he would. When we showed up, it was another nurse who worked at our home. As soon as she saw us walking inside the store, she froze.

We approached the counter, which was totally enclosed behind bulletproof glass, and had the manager hold up the check for us to identify. Sure enough, it'd been stolen. The girl acted confused and left. To our surprise, she drove back to the nursing home to continue working, as if nothing had happened. I called the police from the check-cashing place and they took down the details. Then we all drove back to the home, where I called the nurse into the office and the police officers arrested her. That's when we received yet another surprise.

"What about my son?" she cried.

"What about him?" the officer replied.

"He's in my cousin's car outside."

"What?!" I said, appalled. I ran outside to find a five-year-old boy lying across the backseat playing with a toy. The windows were cracked and it was fairly cool, so he wasn't in danger of heat exposure. Still, this was wrong. The officers asked her about it and she said she didn't have the money for a babysitter. The situation just got worse from there.

The police called their station, which then called Child Protective Services. They took the little boy away, but not before he got to see his mother in handcuffs and placed in a squad car. It was a tough scene to swallow for someone so young.

Because our residents were mostly from the surrounding neighborhood, they were used to events like this. It didn't bother them—just another day. Most of them said they hoped she got out of jail soon. Even though she was stealing, their life experiences told them this sometimes happened and they had to make the best of it. As soon as the police left, life drifted back to normal. I, however, had not grown up in this environment. It took me a while to calm down before starting the search for yet another nurse. It was always something.

In early February we hired Sylvia to replace the nurse headed to prison. It wasn't long before she too became true buddies with the Almond Joys. Soon after that she came into my office and suggested we take some residents up to the Choctaw casino in Durant, Oklahoma. It was just across the Texas border. I blinked several times when I first heard the idea. "How many residents and staff are you thinking would go?"

Sylvia put her finger to her chin and looked up. "Let's see, I would be their nurse and drive the bus. We can fit twelve comfortably, so I guess thirteen. I could take all the meds and DNR sheets, so if they win that big jackpot in the sky, we wouldn't have a problem."

"How long would you stay?"

"Well, we could feed them breakfast here and load them up right afterwards. Then I'd drive up there—it's about an hour and a half—and plop them all down in slot machine heaven. There are places for them to eat there, so they'd be mostly on their own. The ones I'm thinking about taking I'm sure I can handle. They have a little money to gamble with, too."

I thought about my first position at Wellington Hills. They would never allow such a thing. The residents always stayed in one place—that gorgeous facility—and never left unless they had to see a specialty doctor. But with the new spirit of excitement in the home, of energy, of life, I wanted more for my residents. I wanted them to get out and see life, to go to another state, to explore our world and not just see themselves as confined to one location like prisoners.

"Okay. I'll approve the trip, but we need to go over all the details first."

Over the next several days we studied the trip from every angle. I agreed the home would pay for the gas, but not Sylvia. She would go on her day off. I made sure each resident going had enough money and could afford it. Of course, Dale, Ari, and Gracie were going. There was no way they'd be left behind. Ari had very little money, but he still wanted to go. Any of the residents who weren't going gave some money to their trusted buddy to put in a slot machine and see what happened. There were handwritten ledgers everywhere, detailing the bets to be placed for the ones left behind. I shook my head and laughed at it all.

The event took place on a Wednesday, Sylvia's day off. From the time they pulled away to the time they arrived in Choctaw, I was worried. Sylvia called to say they'd arrived safely and that they were all enjoying themselves. At around 7 p.m. she called back and said they were on their way home. I'd decided to stay until they arrived since I knew I'd be too worried at home. When they finally rolled up in front, I had several CNAs ready to help unload the weary gamblers. The first thing I saw as they got off the bus was smiles. Big ones.

"Damn, that was a lot of fun, Administrator," Gracie howled. She seemed to be the most energized of the crew as she rolled around in her chair with an extra burst of energy.

"Quit while you're ahead," Ari added holding up his index finger. "All the best gamblers do."

"And we did," said Dale. "Well, more like quit while we're still alive."

I chuckled. "Was it everything you hoped for?"

"Hell yes," Gracie said. "When can we go back?"

"We'll see. Let me talk to Sylvia first and get a report."

Sylvia stepped into my office. "Any problems?"

"No, things went smoothly. The bellhops helped get everyone off the bus and then loaded us up again when it was time to come home. The residents mostly took care of themselves. After all, they *are* adults."

"Did they gamble a lot?"

She shook her head. "Not particularly. Most of them just liked getting around and seeing the sights. They did have a few drinks, but no one got out of control. Really, it was a good trip."

I was thrilled. The residents who went were very happy and the ones who didn't spent the next few days sucking every detail from the memory banks of the ones who did. For once in Jones-Simms' history we had something Wellington Hills didn't. And for some reason, that thrilled me.

I was about to complete my second year at Jones-Simms and did a self-assessment of my performance. One thing I reflected on was the staff. In the beginning they were inflexible, disloyal, and sometimes rude. Now, they were hardworking, loving, creative and willing to go the extra mile. As I said before, I fully credited the Almond Joys for that. They were the horse that pulled the cart. When they spoke, people listened. Nothing illustrated this more than Bulldozer. He'd been making steady progress ever since his last surgery. Even though Jones-Simms wasn't set up to do much rehab, the staff showed their true colors where his case was concerned. They improvised and created exercises for him to do. And with every lift, one of the Almond Joys was there to document it—usually Ari. He spouted out quotes like, "When the will is ready, the feet are light. Proverbs." "Obstacles are those frightful things you see when you take your eyes off your goal. Henry Ford." And, "The world makes way for the man who knows where he is going. Ralph Waldo Emerson."

Bulldozer responded. He kept saying, "I'm gonna get out of here and go back to work." It was that positive attitude that paid off. Six months after he came to our home he was well enough to leave. The doctors couldn't believe it. They checked him out head to toe and while he didn't look like he could go back to construction, he was able to live with relatives as long as they helped him get around. This would allow him to take advantage of some other social programs that involved better rehabilitation facilities.

The doctors selected the day he could leave and, of course, we threw a big going-away party. It was complete with speeches, music and a lot of tears. We held it over lunch and cooked his favorite foods: baked ham, lima beans, cornbread, and buttered pecan ice cream. He promised to drop by, but I knew the odds of that were slim. He was young and would soon forget this place, much like he wanted to forget his violent assault. I couldn't blame him. I would've done the same.

It was two in the afternoon when Bulldozer hugged everyone and left us for good. I went back to my office to get caught up on some paperwork, while most of the residents dried their eyes and started thinking about a nap. Suddenly I heard a big commotion. I pushed back my chair and said to myself, "What now?"

Stepping out of my office, I walked towards the lobby and noticed several residents in wheelchairs pushing themselves hard to get outside. Six more residents were moving past them faster than I'd ever seen them move. They were all busting through the glass door and heading to the front sidewalk. I hurried my steps and was joined by a nurse who looked worried.

"What's going on?" I asked.

"A knife fight and some of the residents want to get involved!"

"What?!" I yelled, a word that seemed to come out of my mouth over and over.

"Yeah. This could get ugly!" she said running ahead of me.

When I reached the glass door, I saw two combatants with knives slicing at each other as a wave of residents rapidly approached them. I stopped in my tracks and yelled back inside to whoever was listening, "*Call* the police! Call 9-1-1 now!"

Then I foolishly barged through the doors to get involved and perhaps get cut myself. It never crossed my mind that this might be a bad idea.

16

As I raced through the doors, next to me were men in wheelchairs racing at top speed.

"What in the world are you doing?!" I yelled at one of them. "I'm going to break it up. I can handle these two."

The one next to him said, "I'll take the kid in the blue shirt."

"Get back inside!" I screamed unsuccessfully.

The combatants were two high school kids circling each other. Neither one seemed particularly serious about getting sliced open. Of course, with my limited knife-fighting experience, what did I know?

"Cayla!" I yelled, pointing to the male residents in wheelchairs and walkers. Turn these men around and get them back inside." By this time two other CNAs had arrived and were forming a barrier to stop our residents from getting any closer. I was just turning my attention to the combatants when a loud siren sounded, followed by screeching tires. Two officers sprung from their cars and drew their service pistols.

"Drop it now and get on the ground!" Not only did this seem to discourage any additional fighting, but our residents' urge to intervene also ground to a halt. The two kids reluctantly dropped their knives and grabbed some pavement. This was followed by more officers, two sets of handcuffs and eventually, emptiness. By then we had all the residents back inside and were lecturing them about running to a knife fight. That's when Gracie wheeled up and pulled me aside.

"Look Administrator, they still think they're young and capable of stopping a fight. Or maybe they even wanted to get involved. This is what they did all the time before they got trapped in here, when they were much younger. It gets their blood pumping. Get it?"

I knew she was right. Seeing the incident stirred up their testosterone, tricking them into believing they could still take care of things. It was scary to see men in wheelchairs rolling into a knife fight, but it was completely natural for all of them. They'd seen it before and knew they'd see it again.

As for me, I wasn't used to seeing fights of any kind, let alone knife fights. Our facility was filled with folks who came from a world I hadn't known existed. The poverty was shocking. The drugs, alcohol, and violence all worked together to create an unhealthy environment, which of course led many of them to live in facilities like this, if they made it this far. Then there were the Almond Joys. They were the outliers—citizens who didn't belong here. Ari was educated and Dale was an entrepreneur. They both had accumulated money to avoid places like this. That left Gracie, a blue-collar worker. Out of the three, it was easy to see her living here. But she also didn't belong. All three of them were good citizens: people who paid their taxes, voted, stayed informed and tried to do the right thing. Yet here they were at the end of their lives, wards of the state. Their property had been confiscated; their worlds destroyed. I didn't see them running to join the knife fight. They just smiled and survived another day.

A week later I learned about a new fast food joint opening up nearby—Big Dogs. The hot dogs there were supposed to be the best in the city. I'm not a big hot dog eater, but sometimes I needed to get away from the home. One day, before I left to try it out, Dale cornered me.

"Is there any way you could bring a hot dog back for Ari? He loves them." She handed me the money.

"Sure. What does he like on it?"

"Mustard and relish. No onions."

"Okay. I'll be back shortly, but please don't spread it around. I can't be making runs for everyone."

"Now Susan, you know we can keep our mouths shut. Though when Ari gets a hold of that hot dog, his mouth will be moving a lot. That's for sure."

I chuckled. She was probably right.

It took me twenty minutes to get there and sure enough, the place was good. Real good. The fresh buns were steaming and the condiments sizzled when they dropped them on the meat. I ordered a chili-dog with cheese and onions and devoured it in record time. When I got back in line to get Ari's, I actually thought about getting another one for myself, but I was full when it came time to order so I returned with just the one hot dog.

Lunch had already been served and put away when I called Dale and Ari to my office. "Here's your hot dog. The staff can heat it up if you want."

He shook his head and immediately ripped open the foil. Surprisingly, it was still warm. He shoved one end into his mouth and began chomping away, right there in my office. I wasn't overjoyed about this since I was trying to work, but he looked so enraptured I didn't have the heart to throw him out. Instead, I told him and Dale to pull up a chair and enjoy.

Dale had been hunching over farther and farther and was having more trouble walking. Sometimes she used a cane. This time, though, she slid gingerly into the chair.

"Susan, what about planning a trip to the ballpark. Ari loves baseball and studies all the statistics. He'd be thrilled to go." Ari nodded with his mouth full.

"Hmmm. We did plan that trip to Choctaw. And a lot of the residents attended Mr. G's funeral with no hiccups. Why not? Let me get together with the staff and see what we can do. Maybe we can get some cheap tickets."

"That would be wonderful!"

Ari had finished his hot dog by now and was able to spit out the words, "Never let the fear of striking out get in your way. Babe Ruth."

I chuckled. "Okay, Ari. I'll see if we can strike out of here and go to a game."

Dale clapped her hands. "He'd be so excited. It would be like old times."

Ari had a mustard smile from ear to ear. I handed him a tissue, then got busy planning a trip to the ballpark.

It turns out it wasn't that difficult. The Texas Rangers have ticket packages for groups exactly like ours. With the spare money the residents had in their accounts and a little from our activities budget, we were able to set up a fantastic event. So many residents wanted to go that we had to find a larger bus. We managed to scrounge up a raggedy one that would hold everyone plus three CNAs, Cayla, Beth and myself. The bus was rundown, but no one complained. In fact, they sang songs the entire way, like they were children going to summer camp. It was delightful.

The day was very warm, which was comfortable for older people. It was a noon make-up game on a Monday—the perfect time to go. It wasn't that crowded, so the residents got to move around without feeling pressed in. The stadium had an area for us to congregate and even provided snacks and bottled water. Ari, along with several other residents, went directly to the concession stand and ordered some ballpark dogs. That put them in heaven. When I saw a few residents order beers, I looked the other way. After all, it was their life. And it wasn't illegal. I made sure we kept an eye on them. I didn't want anyone getting drunk because an elderly drunk person is a serious injury waiting to happen.

During the fifth inning they flashed a sign on the big screen: "Welcome to the Jones-Simms Nursing Center." This got everyone clapping and congratulating each other like we'd just won the lottery.

When they had a race with three costumed runners, we got to actually play the lottery, though the people who selected the winner didn't get anything other than a pat on the back.

As for our seats, we were far down the third base line—mostly in the outfield. I think if the game hadn't have been a make-up, we would've been off behind right field somewhere. Thankfully, it was and these seats allowed a few fouls balls to come our way. It was hilarious watching some of the men act like they could actually catch one. One resident, Mr. Yellen, had contracture—a condition where the muscles and joints lock up. His hands were constantly in a v-shape over his chest and his ball cap was on sideways. Even so, the entire game he kept yelling, "I want a fly ball!" It was both funny and beautiful to see him thoroughly enjoying himself.

Ari sat in the front row watching the strategy and making notes. Between innings, he studied the official program treating it like a Bible, holding it close to his chest. At the end of the game, fireworks exploded over the scoreboard celebrating the Rangers' win. That was our cue to load the gang back on the bus (with the kind help of the stadium staff and service elevators). Even though a good time was had by all, more than three hours of peanuts, turkey legs, heat, nachos, and the occasional beer caused heavy eyes among our adventurers. In fact, most of the residents were snoring on the ride back. Even I drifted off.

The next day the home was abuzz with memories of the game. Everyone who had attended recounted the events for those who didn't go. When those left behind lost interest, the gamers went over everything once more with their fellow gamers. Since many had memory issues, it was like living through it all over again. Then there was Ari. He poured over his score sheet and the game program like there was some hidden secret between the pages. Every now and then he licked his lips, no doubt recalling the mustard and relish on the hot dogs. I was so grateful Dale had suggested it. A trip to the ballpark had to be something we put on the calendar at least once a year. I was going to make sure of that.

A few days later life was back to normal and the only sign of the big event was several pages of the baseball program tacked to the walls here and there like trophies. I walked past the recreation room and saw a bunch of residents watching something on TV. I assumed it was a baseball game, but I was wrong.

"What's going on?" I asked.

"The hurricane!" Gracie said. "It's going to hit New Orleans and it's gonna be awful."

"We're five hundred miles away. Thank goodness we're not going to be affected."

"A thousand fibers connect us with our fellow man," Ari said. "One pebble in a small pond creates many ripples."

He had a look like he knew something I didn't. I figured the rest of the residents just needed something to be captivated with. Still, I wondered what he could know.

Five days later

"Hello, Billy. How are you doing?" I held the phone away from my ear while he coughed up a lung.

"Okay. Listen, you know that Katrina thing?"

"Yes, of course." There had been nothing else but that on television. The devastation was horrific.

"Yeah, well the government moved all the nursing home residents out of New Orleans to temporary shelters and since they're not going back, they're looking to put them in nursing homes in North Texas. Our outfit got first crack at the bunch, so I can send a mess of 'em to you. How many beds do you have open right now?"

"Fourteen."

More coughing. "Okay, I'm gonna ship over fourteen Cajuns for you to take care of. The feds are picking up the tab for this right now. I'll have the girls send you the paperwork and RUG rates. This is kind of a screwy deal, though. We still have to go through the state while the feds have agreed to pay the RUG rates we've set here at corporate. Got it?"

"Wow, that's wonderful! We'll be full for the first time. When are they coming?"

"I don't know. I'm gonna call right now and have the feds fax you a list of their names and medical requirements. Okay?"

"No problem. I'll call a staff meeting and get on it."

A deep, death-inducing cough. "Listen, some of these poor souls have been through hell. They've been crapping in hallways in the Superdome, seen gators crapping in their homes, been in temporary shelters resembling jails and God knows what else. And you know how old folks like a routine and familiar surroundings. So plan on rolling out the ole red carpet for them."

"Don't worry, we'll take care of them." I was getting more excited by the minute.

"Oh, and one more thing. Pop the top off some of those meds and have them ready. Some of these folks are pretty spazzed out. Okay? They could use a Halcyon holiday."

"Sure," I chuckled. "I'll get Dr. Lowery warmed up and ready to prescribe—if medically necessary, of course."

"Of course, but I think it'll be medically necessary." Another bout of extended, extreme coughing. I went ahead and hung up, assuming corporate would let me know if he died.

My mind was spinning. For the first time we'd be completely full. This had been my main goal from day one. Now, on my first admin job, I was finally ringing the 100% occupancy bell. It was like winning a marathon.

I immediately called the staff together. Once the news sunk in they picked up their pads and pens and wrote down everything they needed to do to make this a smooth transition. Someone was going to make sure all the beds were clean and ready to be slept in. Another was going to be working on the food supply and have extra plates and silverware ready. Beth was planning a welcoming party like we did when the thirteen came over from Warm Heart. The nurses would make sure the meds were ready whenever Dr. Lowery examined the new arrivals and prescribed some happy pills (if necessary, of course). And I would talk to the residents to let them know what was about to happen. My first visit, though, would be with the Almond Joys.

"You're saying we need to be ready to handle the Cajuns?" Gracie shifted a little in her wheelchair, chewing over the news.

"Yes. You three are the leaders of this home. Just like when you were welcomed here, I need you to welcome these poor folks. They've been through so much."

"Yeah," said Gracie. "I remember that welcome, the one where they wanted to kick us out. That's the one you're talking about, right?"

"No, the one I'm talking about is where we welcomed you at the front door with open arms. Remember that? That's what we need to do now. Can I count on you to help me?"

"Yes," Dale said. "We'll make sure they're welcomed and assimilated into our little society here. Do you have their names yet?"

"Yes, my corporate office faxed them over."

"Good. If you'll provide them to me, we'll get their rooms assigned according to sex and start designing special name plates for them. Perhaps we could get the artists among us to design some familiar New Orleans-themed artwork. What's their team there?"

"The Saints," Gracie added. "Yeah, give us the list. Times a-wastin'."

I handed them the list. "Thank you all very much. This is a good thing you're doing."

They turned to leave when Ari stopped and looked around. "Life is divided into three terms—that which was, that which is and that which will be. William Wordsworth."

"Thank you, Ari," I said, unsure of his exact meaning. "I'll keep that in mind, along with all of us being connected. I understand now what you were saying a few days ago about the ripples in the pond. Something far away has now affected us."

He managed a smile and closed the door as he left. Once I had my office to myself, I alternated between excitement and nervousness. This would push us to the max. Would my staff be able to handle it? I sure hoped so.

My phone rang around nine the next morning. "Susan, they're here!" I slammed down the receiver and ran to the front entrance. There parked at the curb was an old Greyhound bus. I straightened my dress and calmly walked outside to greet a woman coming towards me.

"Hi there! And welcome to the Jones-Simms . . ." She cut me off.

"Save the greeting for them," she said pointing with a thumb over her shoulder at the bus. "Believe me, they're going to need it."

I watched as the bus driver lifted up the sides, revealing dozens of military-style canvas bags. Behind those were wheelchairs, walkers and cots. Lots of cots.

"Sign here," she said, thrusting a clipboard at me. I looked down at the form listing the new residents.

"Hey, this isn't the fourteen we were scheduled to receive."

"Tell me something I don't already know."

"But I don't understand. This shows we're receiving fifty-three people. Why does it say that?"

"Because that old bus has only fifty-five freaking seats. I told Grinder I wasn't going to make this trip without help, so he stuck me with Doofus Junior over there. Otherwise there'd be fifty-four people on the list."

I gazed at the young man helping the driver remove the luggage. "I don't understand. Billy said we're getting fourteen. Who's Grinder?"

"He's my boss. Look lady, I've been on the road since Katrina hit. I've gotten maybe ten hours of sleep, including the hour I just snagged on the bus in some godforsaken place called Balch Springs. Have you heard of Balch Springs?"

"Yes, that's a suburb of Dallas. But I don't understand—we're only supposed to get fourteen."

"Here's the deal lady. Either sign this clipboard or we'll load 'em up and take 'em back to Balch Springs. I don't really care. We have another two hundred waiting for us there."

"But how are we going to care for fifty-three?" This wasn't registering with her.

"I don't know, but I do know we have all these cots my boss had us load up. So do you want to sign or not?" Now she was clearly upset.

I shook my head. "I don't understand," was all I could manage. I had a state license. I couldn't jeopardize that. Plus, there was no way we had the staff or facility for fifty-three people. This was crazy. No, it was insane.

"Hey! Stop unloading. We have an issue here. Wait a sec." She turned back to me. "Lady, I don't have all day. Either sign or write reject on the signature line and we'll get out of here. In fact, the more I look around, the more it looks like a good place to die."

I stood there not believing this turn of events. It felt like a good friend was asking me to just carry some cocaine over to another person. It was that simple. All I had to do was take a hold of the bag and walk it over to the waiting addict, or in this case, sign the form.

I stared at the clipboard. I knew our facility was not rated for this many people. I was about to break the law. I looked back at the two men standing beside the bus. They had already stopped unloading and the driver was lighting a cigarette. I stared back at the clipboard and thought hard. This was so wrong. What I should do was go back inside and call Billy. He would straighten this out. That's what I *should* do. Instead, I took her pen and signed my name on the form.

She jerked the clipboard away and studied my signature. "Hey, you need to date it right here."

"Oh, sorry." I put the date next to my signature. No sense in having any confusion about the exact date I lost my license. The next thing I knew, cots were streaming into my home side by side with wheelchairs loaded with dazed people. Behind them were the walkie-talkies, all of whom looked like zombies. They'd lost everything. The only good news was that they hadn't started with much. Sometimes that makes losing everything a little more palatable.

Forty-five minutes later, the air brakes hissed and the old bus eased away with Doofus Junior and some person who had never told me her name. The devastation from Katrina had come to my very doorstep and it wasn't pretty.

17

Two days later cots lined the recreation room, the lobby and every square inch of floor space other than the food prep and dining area. I made a conscious decision to keep the dining room open. Meals were too important to mess with. The current residents needed at least one place that hadn't changed.

For meal service, though, we were literally getting hammered. First, we were way short of food. Our staff went on a buying spree to cover us for the next few days, but I wasn't sure even that would hold us. Next, we decided to serve the invalids in their rooms rather than haul them to the dining area. It saved the overworked CNAs time and saved us dining room space. Finally, we had to have two rounds of seating at each meal. With a shortage of tables and chairs, there was no other way to do it. That made each meal a major event, lasting twice as long as before. Paper plates were now the norm, since we didn't have enough dishes. It was tough. My entire staff was stressed. I was stressed. Minor arguments turned into major blow-ups and we hadn't even made forty-eight hours. I could only imagine what a month of this looked like.

I watched the food prep staff furiously setting tables for lunch. They'd just cleared away the breakfast trays and had thirty minutes before they had to serve the regular residents and a select few new arrivals. I was about to pitch in and start helping when our receptionist caught my attention. "Hey Susan, there are two people here to see you. I think they're with the state."

"Okay, I'll be right there." I knew Billy had been working with the feds to see if the state would take control of these people or do something else with them. These two were probably here for that. I straightened myself up and made my way to the lobby.

Standing behind the receptionist's desk were two nicely dressed bureaucrats—a middle-aged male and a youngish female. The female was busy snapping photos of the people in the cots while the man furiously scribbled notes on a pad. They looked serious, which made me happy. I wanted everyone to know the hell we were going through. Hopefully these two could open up the pipeline and get some of these people placed in other homes.

"Hello, I'm Susan Hodges, the administrator for the Jones-Simms Nursing Center. How can I help you?"

"I'm Lanny Tiller and this is Jane Smith. We're from DADS. Did you say your name is Susan Hodges?"

"Yes, it is," I said as he wrote it down on his pad.

"And what is your license number?"

"57256941. Why?" I was starting to lose that happy feeling.

"We have to document everything properly so when the board takes your license we can be sure it's the proper one."

"What?!" I said raising my hands. "What are you talking about?"

He pulled out a form and ran his finger down it. "Gee, let's see. There are more than twenty people sleeping in your lobby and we haven't even started down the hall where I see ten more. This here says you're rated by the state for 115 beds. All these people are lying in cheap cots. They have no closet or bathroom and the square footage requirement is nonexistent. So what are *you* talking about?"

I was about to panic when I broke into a big smile. "I get it. This is a big joke. Well congratulations, you got me. You really got me."

"Oh we're gonna get you all right. You need to take us on an inion through your facility right now."

He was dead serious. If this was a joke, these folks were great actors. "Can I see some identification please?"

They whipped out business cards and plastic badges. I studied everything. "So you really are with the state?"

"Yes, of course. Do you really expect us to believe you think this is a joke? People on cots all over the floor. This is outrageous! How you got a license, I don't know."

Now I knew they were serious. "Did someone complain?"

"No, but what does that matter? We just happened to be scheduled for your yearly survey this morning and we walked in to find this! Clearly you're not in compliance. Your 2567 will be very long indeed." He handed me the standard forms to post on all entrances that the state was in the facility and anyone with a question could speak directly with them.

"Oh, I see. This is a random event. You folks weren't sent by the feds to start moving them out, right?"

"No, we're not with the feds. I said we're with the state." I could see he was wondering if I was on drugs.

"Look, the feds begged us to take all these people. They're from Katrina. You know, New Orleans? They had to evacuate. This is just a temporary deal, an emergency. We're not keeping them long term. We can't even fit them all here. They arrived just two days ago."

"Katrina? All these?"

"Well, fifty-three actually. We had fourteen beds open and those are filled with Katrina victims, too."

They hesitated for a moment and glanced at each other. Then the man spoke again. "We weren't told about any of this. We're here to do a yearly survey of your facility and that's all we know. Now please show us around so we can get on with it."

"Wait a minute, I need to call someone." I left them standing there as I ran down the hall towards my office.

"We'll start without you, ma'am," he called out. I closed my door anyway.

Snatching up the phone, I dialed corporate. When Billy picked up, I was out of breath. "DADS is here! They just happened to pick this day of all the days to do their yearly survey."

"Aww shit! No way we can let this go down. They'll give us so many deficiencies and fines we'll be out of business." I noticed he didn't mention anything about me losing my license. "Susan, I'm on it. Stall them all you can."

I raced back to find them snapping more photos and taking notes. By now the Almond Joys had heard about what was going on. I motioned for them to come into the laundry room for a moment. When they were inside, I closed the door tightly.

"Look, I need you to slow these two down, keep them from leaving. They're supposed to do a survey which lasts a week, but they may just take some photos and leave. They may also call in an out-of-compliance emergency. Then we'll have state people crawling all over us. My boss is calling the big bosses right now to stop them. Can you figure out a way to distract them?"

Ari stiffened his posture and held up an index finger. "Delay is preferable to error. Thomas Jefferson."

Dale patted him on the back. "Don't worry, Susan. We'll take care of it."

Gracie looked up at her. "What's the plan?"

"You're going to say you need to show them something and take them out to the patio. You know those plantings we were joking about last week?"

Gracie grinned. "Got it! I'll be the crazy and you'll be the straight."

"Exactly. That'll buy us maybe twenty minutes."

"Good," I said. "You folks have a plan. Do what you can." I had no idea what they were talking about and went back to the lobby.

A few minutes later I had an urgent call on line two. It was Syp.

"Hey Syp, did you hear what's going on?"

"Yeah, I just need their names."

I gave it to him.

"I'll call you back." *Click.*

I went to the lobby, knowing the receptionist would be the first to get any calls for me. That's when I saw Mr. Tiller and Ms. Smith moving briskly down the hall towards me. Mr. Tiller was talking into a cell phone.

"No, they're all up and down the hall. They're everywhere. I have photos! . . . I've never seen so many violations. I don't care if they're Katrina victims. They deserve respect. This is almost as bad as the Superdome . . . Yes, I get it. We're leaving now, but that won't stop me from protesting this . . . Oh you'll get my memo, too. I'm documenting this for sure. Goodbye."

He closed the phone and stared hard at me. "You win this time, but we'll be back. I don't know who you called, but they're going to see these photos."

"I understand, sir. Have a nice day." I gave him a big, wide smile.

He spun around and left in a huff, his sidekick right alongside. I thought, how wonderful it would be to live in a world that was all black and white. On or off. Right or wrong. No need for flexibility, decisions, or compromise. A world like that wouldn't require anyone to think. You're going one mile over the speed limit, here's your ticket. Never mind if it's an ambulance carrying your mother to the hospital. Simple. Clean. Computer-like. Not something I want to be a part of.

A few minutes later I found the Almond Joys laughing up a storm. "How did it go?"

"Great!" Dale said. "Gracie fooled them out on the patio. She went to show them where the other residents were buried. Then I came along and explained that she wasn't right in the head. Afterwards I took them to see some other 'violations,' like the artwork hanging on the walls and toilet paper rolls almost out. By the time they realized we were wasting their time, the man's cell phone rang and poof! They were gone."

I laughed. "I can't thank you three enough. I seem to keep saying that, don't I?"

Dale nodded. "We know you're taking care of us, even though we don't belong here."

"Yeah," Gracie chimed in. "You've got our back. We know that."

Ari held his finger up again. "Government's first duty is to protect the people, not run their lives. Ronald Reagan."

"That's right," Dale said. "We know you'll make sure nothing happens to us. That's why we make sure nothing happens to you."

"Listen, you have my promise. I'm not going to let anybody mess with you. Besides, I'd have to start doing my job instead of letting you three do it."

We all had a good laugh followed by hugs and I went back to my office. No sooner had I sat down than the phone rang. It was Syp.

"Thank you for making that call," I said. "It was perfect. I loved seeing those two leave in a huff."

"I had to go all the way up to the top on this one. But listen, while I got you on the phone, do not breathe a word to the probate courts of all these Katrina victims here, especially to Ms. Stahl. Understand?"

"Of course, but it's hard to keep some things under wraps. I mean, we have fifty-three people here."

"I know, but don't do any media interviews or let the word get out that they're here. If the courts find out, they'll come and snatch some of them for their program. Got it?"

"Wow, are those people really that desperate?"

"You have no idea. Just make sure you have the $45 in on time for each resident, okay?"

"We do. Melva's on top of that. She doesn't like getting calls from Nala."

"Good. I've got to run." *Click.*

With that the state was off my case and all I had to do was figure out how we were going to manage all of these people.

Three weeks went by and the pressure of overcrowding had eased. The feds, along with our help, found relatives to take some of the victims and nursing homes to take the others. It seemed every day a bus rolled up and took one or two more off to try to pick up the pieces of their lives. Eventually we were back to one meal setting and the CNAs had time to get the invalids out of their rooms and into the dining room. Carlos had worked triple time and seriously needed some time off. Most of his days had been spent unclogging toilets and snaking lines. The large amount of residents had overworked our ancient sewer system. The only blessing was the lack of rain. Flooding during these last few weeks would've been a complete disaster.

Alisha hired two more workers for her food service team and that really made a difference. Fortunately, the nurses and CNAs worked well through this entire ordeal with a heaping dose of the Almond Joys. The three spent all of their free time calming folks down and making them feel welcome. I couldn't imagine what this all would've been like without them.

The only sad incident happened during the second week of the newcomers. A man from New Orleans was standing in the hall talking to another Katrina victim when he had a heart attack. A nurse was right with him instantly, telling me to call for an ambulance. When I got back they were performing chest compressions on him. I could only stand there with my hands to my face. The incident reminded me of how powerless I'd been when my husband had died of a heart attack in our driveway all those years ago. I wasn't home at the time, but the helplessness of the entire scene had me frozen. Like then, there was nothing I could to do to save this man. He died right there on the floor, right in front of me.

For the next several days I had trouble concentrating and sleeping. I only snapped out of it when I reminded myself that despite my controlling nature, I was in control of nothing. It was a tough pill to swallow.

Another situation we had to deal with was Mr. Jenkins. He was a nice man with dementia who was nearing his end. He was on the probate court's program, so part of his money went to pay the $45 each month. His family told me that he'd had enough money at some point and should've done better than our place, but for some reason the money was gone. I heard more than one of the family members curse Mr. Winters, the court assigned guardian. He was an odd fellow who rarely came by and seemed almost sick each time he did. But suddenly, Mr. Winters was showing up a lot. He was looked vibrant, healthy and interested. Maybe he'd awoken from his bureaucratic coma and decided to start doing his job.

When hospice came to take over Mr. Jenkins' care, things got sticky. A daughter was fighting with her two older brothers about the hospice care. I tried to stay on the fringes of the argument, but was soon dragged into it. The daughter wanted all lifesaving measures taken. She was not ready to let go of her father and was upset with our nurses and doctor for not keeping him alive longer. The brothers, on the other hand, didn't want to see him suffer. They were ready to let him go. Our staff had to break up their arguments more than once. It was turning ugly.

Outnumbered, the daughter enlisted the help of Mr. Winters. He agreed with the daughter and wanted Mr. Jenkins to live as long as *inhumanly* possible. Why? I have no idea. I couldn't imagine his cut of the $45 was the deciding factor. It was interesting to note that Melva was receiving a weekly call from Nala Stahl, ensuring that the guardian had been there. For some reason she also was interested. To make matters worse, the doctors had paperwork signed by both sides of the family. The brothers had executed DNRs (papers clearly stating 'Do Not Resuscitate'), while the daughter had signed counter forms. The hospice doctor was trying to administer soothing drugs to help Mr. Jenkins, while the main physician had to make the appearance that he was trying to keep Mr. Jenkins alive. I think all of us professionals were hoping Mr. Jenkins would make it easy on us and give up the fight. For me, I thought the whole affair ironic: a man who'd spent his entire life working for the court (he'd had a long career as a court clerk) was now being managed by the court.

The Almond Joys tried their best to keep everything calm, yet even they weren't able to manage the anger in his family. And Mr. Jenkins' dementia prevented any rational conversation. Once though, Gracie happened to have another dementia resident with her and they stopped in to see Mr. Jenkins. Surprisingly, he suddenly came alive and began talking with the female resident. Gracie rolled away and let them have at it.

A few hours later, she came to tell me about it. "I watched them talk for a while—it was like they understood each other. Right now Dale and Ari have Mr. Gomez talking with Mrs. Nichols. Dale said they seem to understand each other, too. Do you think that's possible?"

"You know, I've never thought about it. I guess it's possible. Are you saying there's a certain frequency they communicate on, one we don't have access to?"

"I don't know about that, but Mr. Jenkins seems to understand. And he was interested, which is more than I've seen from him in the past month. Normally he's pretty dead, if you know what I mean."

I met with the staff and discussed this phenomenon with them. A few CNAs and nurses agreed. They'd seen it before. I directed Beth to start having activities with just the dementia residents and asked everyone to observe their behavior whenever they could. I didn't want to create something that wasn't there, but if we were onto something, I wanted to pursue it.

Mr. Jenkins finally died, and when he did the angst between the siblings reached its climax. At one point, we had to escort the daughter from the building. What happened after they left, I never learned. I assumed it was lawsuits and a fractured family for life. It was sad to see a family ripped apart by something that's going to happen to all of us.

A few days later the Almond Joys appeared in my office. "To whom do I owe the pleasure of this visit?"

"Me, I guess," Gracie said, banging into the chairs. "We need to talk."

When all three of them were situated around my desk, I leaned back and waited to hear the latest request for a new club. Or maybe it was a toilet for Mr. Henson. Or more flowers for the patio. "Well?" I said. "What is it?"

Gracie cleared her throat and gripped the arms of the wheelchair. She glanced at both Dale and Ari, receiving a nod back from each of them. Taking in a deep breath and slowly letting it out, she finally told me the news: "Administrator, we want to go home."

18

I sat up straight having no idea what they had in mind. "Home?" I said weakly. "And where is that?"

"Where we used to live," Dale replied. "We want to go back in time. Is that too much to ask?"

I coughed. "Back in time?"

Gracie looked determined. "Yeah, you know, like you take us to where we used to live and let us see the places we're from one more time."

"Oh, I think I get it. You want to drive by these places? Sort of a trip down memory lane?"

"Exactly," Dale said. "We want to go to some familiar places. Gracie wants to go to her old diner. I want to drive by my store. Ari wants to drive by his house, the one he lived in forever."

I relaxed. "Okay, and when do you want to do this?"

Gracie didn't hesitate. "As soon as possible. When Mr. Jenkins died, we realized we're gonna be joining him soon. We may even get dementia too. Can it be done?"

I owed these three big time, but my mind was still calculating all the variables. Needing a nurse. Injury. Other residents wanting to take a trip, too. There was a lot to think about. "Why don't I check on it and get back with you?"

Gracie's grip tightened on her wheels. "Look, you don't need to check on nothing. Why can't we three just pile into your SUV and take off?"

I hadn't thought about *me* taking them. Sure, I knew her wheelchair would fit in the rear. Dale sometimes needed a walker. That would fit in there, too. All Ari needed was a cane. I could belt two in the backseat and one in the front. But what was I thinking? Taking residents around for a ride wasn't normal. Perhaps it wasn't even allowed.

"This is a new idea. I've never thought about something like this before. Can I please have a day to consider it?"

Dale touched Gracie's shoulder. "Let her have some time. But honestly, Susan, we don't need a bus with a CNA. If you could drive us, that would be all we need. I can't tell you how much it would mean to us."

"Could you three provide me with the addresses of where you want to go? That might make it easier."

"We'll do that. Come on gang, we have an art class starting up soon. We'd better get moving."

When Ari stood up, he raised his finger again. "If it's important to you, you'll find a way. If not, you'll find an excuse."

The other two nodded and left with Ari. I had to admit, I was seriously thinking about granting their request without even asking permission from corporate. I could apologize later, if need be.

I looked up the addresses of where they wanted to go and calculated the entire trip would take barely a half a day. If I did it on a weekend and not on company time, I wouldn't have to leave the home or my job during a weekday when something might happen. That would be too big of risk (not to mention, wrong). Still, there were risks with this trip. If they were injured in my care I could be in big trouble. Or if they took off. Or refused to come back. Any number of things could happen. Still, this wasn't a prison. If they had relatives who could take them out, they were certainly allowed to leave. It was their right. The more I thought about it, the more I wanted to do it. A day later, I went to find them.

We had set up a pie bar in the dining room (yet another idea of the Almond Joys). The first time they suggested it was on National Pie Day in January. It had been so much fun we decided to do it once a quarter. Alisha had the staff whip up an extravagant array of pies: coconut cream, apple, pecan, chocolate, cherry, banana cream, pumpkin, and key lime. As always, the residents were excited. I spotted my three amigos sitting at a table enjoying their pie and moved towards them. Out of the corner of my eye, I saw Shanda, one of our nurses, take a piece of lemon meringue pie away from Mr. Reynolds.

"Oh, I just wanted one piece," he moaned. "It's been so long since I had some."

Shanda placed it back on the main table. "You're a diabetic. You know you can't be having pie."

I stopped in my tracks. "Shanda, can I see you in my office, please?"

She looked at me and knew she was in trouble. I walked over to the pie table. "Here Mr. Reynolds, have a piece of pie. Eat all you want."

His eyes watered up as his shaking hand grabbed the plate. "Oh thank you, ma'am! Thank you so much."

I took Shanda into my office, and before I could speak she started in. "Look, he's a diabetic and he's going to need a huge shot of insulin in one hour. Do you know that?"

"Of course I know that. Do we have the insulin?"

"Yes, but . . ."

"Do we have the needles?"

"Yes, but . . ."

"Then what's the problem?"

"I'm going to be the one who has to give it to him."

I frowned. "Are you getting paid while you stick him with a needle?"

"Yes, but I have other things to do. Besides, he could literally kill himself with all that sugar."

"Yes, he may. But in Texas he has that right. If he wants to go into a coma, he has that right. We're getting paid to make sure his rights are protected. In my house, if he wants four pieces of pie, you'll shoot him with all the insulin he needs. If he dies today, so be it. It's his right."

"But . . ."

"No, I don't want to hear anything more. If we followed your logic we'd stop giving all of them food and water just so we don't have to clean their diapers. They live here! This is their home. *We* are the guests in it. And guests don't tell owners how much pie they can have. Got it?"

"Yes, ma'am."

"Good, now let's get back to work."

I was pretty steamed and walked around for a few minutes making sure everyone who wanted pie got it. It wasn't until things were winding down that I signaled for the Almond Joys to come to my office.

"You're not gonna keep us from our pie, are you?" Gracie said sarcastically.

"Are you talking about pie as in food, or pie as in your trip?"

"What do you think?"

"I think we will go on your memory lane tour this Saturday morning. I'll pick you up at the front lobby after breakfast. You be there and have everything you need to be gone for the day. I'll check you out."

Dale clapped her hands while Ari's face was lit up. Gracie, though, was unfazed. She probably knew what my answer would be.

"Any questions?" I asked.

They shook their heads.

"Good. I'll see you then and please keep this to yourselves. I don't need to be taking the entire home with me." I knew that when the others found out, many of them would want trips down their own memory lanes as well. If that happened, I'd just have to deal with it. One thing I was sure of though, this was going to be a unique experience.

I pulled away from the Jones-Simms Nursing Center with my three buddies. By now they were more like relatives, especially Dale. The women were in the backseat and Ari was in the front; we were going to his place first. "Are you all excited?"

"Very," piped Dale.

Ari nodded. Sometimes he preferred to make gestures rather than talk. I drove the rest of the way without saying much, but when I pulled down Ari's street I saw his body stiffen. He gripped the armrest and stared intently at each house. I slowed down.

His eyes seemed fixed on a one-story, ranch-style house with a brick exterior. A car sat in the driveway, a driveway with 50 years of cracks in it and probably a story for each one. The brick looked like it'd been painted over several times. Two large trees threw sweeping canopies over the roof and front porch, keeping it in perpetual shade. This design had done away with traditional porches, the kind where you could sit and visit with neighbors. The mailbox was right next to the front door, making sure the occupants never had to venture out more than two feet.

"Is this it, Ari?"

He nodded, though I'd already guessed the answer from the look in his eyes.

"Would you like to get out?"

He was already unfastening the seatbelt and reaching for the door. I twisted around to the backseat. "Do you ladies want to join him?"

Dale said, "We'll stay here and see what he does. If he needs me, I'll get out."

I helped Ari around the car and over the curb. He stood there shaking. I could tell he wanted to go up the sidewalk to the front door, but there was no need—the door suddenly opened with a middle-aged man eyeing us warily. He was dressed in workout clothes and obviously about to leave. "Can I help you folks?" he asked.

"I'm Susan Hodges." I left Ari and walked towards the man. "We're from a nursing home on the other side of town. The man behind me used to live here. We're taking a trip down memory lane, so to speak."

"Oh. Well I can't let you inside because I have to go right now. But you can stand in the yard and walk around to the side of the fence. Roscoe is pretty friendly, though I wouldn't try to go in the backyard."

"We won't and thank you for your kindness. We won't be long. He just wants to relive some memories."

"How long ago did he live here?"

"About five years ago."

"We bought it out of foreclosure about then. Hey, that reminds me. There was a baseball glove we found tucked away in the garage. Actually, I have it in my trunk. I've been meaning to give it to some kid but never found the right one. Would he like it back?"

"That would be wonderful. It might even be his."

Ari's eyes opened wide. The man rummaged through the trunk for a moment before declaring, "Here it is." He handed Ari the glove, who turned it over and over before slipping it over his hand. Sure enough, the glove was his.

Ari proclaimed, "There are only two seasons, winter and baseball. Bill Veeck."

I smiled at the man. "He likes to speak in quotes."

The man nodded. "I'm glad I could return that. Now, if you'll excuse me, I've got to get going. Take care."

I waved at him. "Thanks for your kindness, sir. Really."

Ari called out, "I would like to thank you from the bottom of my heart, but for you my heart has no bottom." The man chuckled and drove off, leaving us standing in his yard.

"Ari, would you like to look around?"

He nodded and went to the chain link fence to gaze at the backyard. A beagle came sauntering over, wagging his tail. He decided pretty quickly that we were harmless. I stayed back and let Ari take in all he wanted. After several minutes passed, Ari sighed and began shuffling back to the car, tears streaming down his face.

As I got back in the car, Dale spoke up. "Susan, a playground where Ari used to throw the ball around with the neighborhood kids is a few blocks away. Could we drive by that, just so he could take a look?"

"Sure."

She gave me directions and I pulled up to a large park that had a backstop, soccer goalposts and a nice playground for smaller kids. A few people were out walking their dogs, but otherwise the park was deserted. Ari rolled down the window and stared. He still had his baseball glove on and hit it several times with his other hand. Eventually, he wiped his tears and rolled up the window. I reached over and patted his leg. "I hope it was a good trip for you, Ari. I really do."

He nodded and smiled. "Happiness will never come to those who fail to appreciate what they already have."

"Amen to that," I said. "Amen."

We sat in silence for a while, letting Ari work through his emotions. When the time seemed right, I checked my map and started towards our next destination: Dale's antique store.

The address I'd been given was a strip center on a fairly busy street, yet it wasn't a prime location for major stores. It didn't even have an anchor. Instead, it was simply a collection of destination stores that needed cheap rent to make the numbers work. Perfect for an antique store.

"Right over there, Susan," Dale said, her voice rising with anxiety. I followed her instructions and stopped in front of a fabric store. She seemed stunned.

"Do you want to get out?"

Without an answer, the car door opened. I got out and helped her move towards the entrance, leaving her walker behind. I was a little worried about this, but she seemed steady enough. Though the lights inside were already on, the door plaque said it didn't open until ten. I looked at my watch. That was ten minutes away. Now I could see a few tears trickling down Dale's face. This was the store that had been ripped away from her by the probate court, the guardian and her daughter. We stood there while she gazed inside at the fixtures, obviously recognizing a few of them.

The fabric store was sandwiched between a spice store and an insurance company. Both spaces had turned over in the six years since she'd lost everything, so she didn't know them either. She was taking it all in, trying to decide how she felt about the whole thing. When ten o'clock finally arrived, a lady came and opened the door.

"Welcome. Can I help you find anything?"

"Yes," I said. "Years ago, Dale here used to run an antique store from this very spot. We're taking a trip down memory lane. Do you mind if we just walk around the store a little?"

"Be my guest."

Dale asked, "How long have you worked here, honey?"

"I've only been working here a year."

"Who owns this store?"

"Ruth Long. I'm sure she'd be happy to talk with you if she were here. But she's out of town, buying more fabric."

Dale walked over to a large shelf fixture. "These used to be mine," she whispered to me. "It sure hurts seeing all this."

"Do you want to leave?"

"No, I'm happy to see it, even though it hurts."

After a few minutes of roaming through the entire store, Dale got the clerk's attention. "Do you mind if I use the restroom?"

"Go ahead. It's in the back, although I guess you know where it is."

"Yes, I do. Thank you kindly."

I was waiting near the checkout counter when Dale reappeared with a smile on her face. "We can go now."

"Thank you, ma'am," I said. "It's been enjoyable for her."

"Yes, thank you again," Dale added.

"Come back anytime."

Once we were in the car, Dale handed me something to look at. "What's this?"

Giddily she said, "I found it just where I left it all those years ago. It was taped next to the wall phone."

I took it from her and studied it closely. It was a business card that read Auntie's Antiques. Directly below was the address and phone number. Then I saw what she was so proud of: Dale Waterson, Proprietor. "Well, I'll be darned. Both you and Ari got a nice memento from your trip down memory lane. What are you going to do with it?"

"I'm going to laminate it in plastic and pin it to my wall. This may seem hard to believe, but that little card is going to remind me each day of the life I used to lead." She started choking up.

"It's okay," Gracie said. "Just let it out." Dale leaned her head on Gracie's shoulder and had a good cry.

I sat there for a few minutes allowing the moment to happen. Then I asked, "Ready to go, Dale?"

"Yes, we can move on. And thanks again for bringing me. I'm sad, but I'm happy too."

"I happy for you. Glad you got what you wanted. Now, we're on to the last stop!"

I was hoping to have them back at the home in time for lunch. Right now, things were looking good. Still, we had to drive to the other side of town taking a full twenty minutes. By the time we got there, it was 10:45 a.m., which was actually perfect for this place.

I pulled up in front. "Okay Gracie, now it's your turn. You ready?"

"Yeah, I'm ready. Let's go."

I got Dale and Ari out of the car first, then worked Gracie's wheelchair into position. Dale motioned for her walker, so I set that up too. When all of us were out and situated we took one long look at the place in front of us: Mama's Diner. I could tell the place had been a popular spot in its day, but the changes in the neighborhood and new restaurants popping up had taken their toll. Still, it was here and so were we. We went inside with Gracie leading the way.

The moment we opened the doors my nose was assaulted by a cacophony of smells: toast, fried eggs, grease, coffee (black and hot).

Gracie wheeled in and was greeted by a waitress. "You can sit wherever you like."

Gracie asked her, "Is Emilio here?"

"Emilio? I don't know him. Does he work here?"

"He used to. Does Sarge still own this place?"

"Sarge? I don't know him either. Let me ask the cook in the back. He's been here longer than me."

I watched her disappear through some swinging doors. The place had four customers—two at the counter and the other two in separate booths. Definitely not the busy time. A minute later, a large black man appeared from the back. Instantly, Gracie recognized him. "Lamar!"

"Gracie? Is that you?"

"Yes! Come on over here and give me a big ole hug."

He bent down and wrapped his muscled arms around her. They embraced for quite a while. It was obvious they'd been very close.

"What are you doing out this way?"

"I'm taking a trip down memory lane. I live in a nursing home now, with these good people behind me. Let me introduce you to them." Wheeling around she said, "This is Ari." The two men shook hands. "This is Dale. And this is Susan, the administrator at the home I live in. She's our tour guide for today."

He shook hands with both of us. "Pleased to meet you folks. Man, Gracie and me go way back. We slung a lot of hash together. We shor' nuff did."

"Lamar always had my back. When I was slowing down, he picked up the slack. I owe him a lot, too much, really." Gracie started choking up.

Lamar patted her on the back. "Hey, hey, none of that in here. This is happy times. Remember?"

"Happy times, yeah. I remember." It was obviously something private amongst themselves. "Does Sarge still own it?"

"Nah, he sold out the year you left. Tanji Farhat owns it now. He's from India. Owns a couple of other joints too. Let's see . . . you left what, eight years ago? I guess I'm the only one left. They just can't get rid of me."

"And well they shouldn't," she said dabbing at her eyes.

"Listen, can I make you folks something to eat? It's on me."

"No way, Lamar. It's on me. And I would love you forever if you'd let me help you cook it."

He studied her wheelchair. "Can you move around in that thing?"

"Sure I can. Remember my sliding stool? I managed."

"Well, I guess it's safe. What are they going to do, fire me? Hell, no one else knows where everything is. Why don't you folks sit down and let Patti take your order. Gracie and I will be working hard in the back to sling it out."

"Get whatever you want," she said. "It's on me."

"If you insist," I said, smiling. "C'mon gang. Let's find a booth."

Patti came and took our order. I wanted some breakfast; both Dale and Ari ordered lunch. Fifteen minutes later the plates arrived, each decorated with unique garnishes. Ari's plate had a smiley face made out of mustard. Dale had several pickles propped up like a teepee. Mine had two small tomatoes with unique carvings. It was very special.

We took our time, savoring our food and lingering over the drinks. It was clear that the enjoyment for Ari and Dale was the fact that they knew Gracie was back there enjoying everything. Sometimes, just seeing your loved ones incredibly happy is the best thing there is.

By 11:45 a.m. more customers had trickled in and more plates were coming out. I was beginning to wonder if Gracie had gotten lost, but she finally she reappeared. Rolling over to our booth, she said, "This has been the best day of my life. Really! I can't tell you how great this was."

"We're happy for you. Do you want to stay here and eat?"

"No, Lamar fixed me up something special back there. I ate it all up so quickly that he put more in a to-go box. And he gave me something else." She held up a small, rusted can opener. "This little can opener has been back there for maybe 30 years. It's punched holes in more cans of milk, oil, and juice than I could ever count. We kept it on a chain and it never needed replacing. You can't ever destroy these things."

It was funny to see how such a seemingly worthless item could be so valuable. "That's wonderful Gracie," I said. "Really, it is."

Dale joined me. "Yes dear, it looks like you had the time of your life."

"I did! I really did."

"Did you get to cook?"

"Well, I cooked each of your meals. Lamar had to reach a few things for me, but I put it all together myself. Was it good?"

"Wonderful!" Dale and I said in unison.

Ari chimed in. "You don't need a silver fork to eat good food. Paul Prudhomme."

Gracie chuckled. "Thanks Ari. Well, I guess it's time to go."

"Do we need to leave a tip?" I asked.

"No, it's already taken care of."

"Okay folks, let's go." We got to our feet and waved goodbye to Patti. Once we were loaded up in the car, I headed back to the Jones-Simms home carrying three good people along with their very heavy hearts.

On Monday, I filled in Melva with the details of the memory lane tour. The stories made her smile. Who wouldn't? It was a joyful and endearing time. I even wondered how other residents would do on such a trip. Before we finished, however, Melva let me know the probate court was auditing us. "They want to make sure we're sending in all the money we're supposed to."

"Boy, they don't want to miss a dime. Do they think we're cheating them?"

"Honestly, I don't know. They may. This 'Nala the Wall' is both rude and condescending. She holds the power of the judge over us constantly. I've heard other homes mail their payment in late or leave off a few $45 fees just to see if they're looking. Sometimes they are and sometimes they aren't. But if you're caught, Nala always threatens to pull residents from a home. It's pretty intimidating."

"Yeah, but she's not going to pull residents from this home. It's too stressful for the resident. Still, remember what Syp says: cooperate and leave them alone. It's like being pulled over by a cop. Keep your hands on the steering wheel and make no sudden movements."

"Believe me, there will be no sudden movements here. Rest assured, we're in good shape."

"Good. We've worked too hard to get this place into the shape it is now. The happiness level here is very high and I don't want to jeopardize that."

We finished our meeting and soon, the duties of the day pushed Nala Stahl and her audit completely out of my mind.

A week later, Gracie's daughter, Mae, was back for a visit. The Almond Joys were holding their reading club, so instead of chatting, Mae joined them as they helped two CNAs and several children read through their lessons. It was amazing to see how much growth and maturity blossomed out of students when they improved their reading skills, especially in the adults. After the club was over, Gracie spent her time with Mae, slipping the homemade necklace on Mae, who made her way to me. "Ms. Hodges, what do you think?" Mae showed off the necklace to me.

"I think it's gorgeous! It looks so good on you."

She beamed. "Mom is going to let me have it one day as an inheritance."

I knew she didn't fully grasp what that meant. "Let's hope that's not for a long time, Mae."

"Don't worry," Dale interrupted. "We're keeping an eye on her, making sure she takes her meds and all that. She's going to be around for a long time."

Mae gave me a hug. "Take good care of my mom. She's all I got."

"Mae, your mother actually takes care of me. So does Dale and Ari, for that matter. They mean so much to this place!"

Mae was still beaming. Even her simple mind could understand that.

"Now you folks enjoy yourself. I have to get some work done." They were gabbing up a fest the moment I left. I felt confident that if Gracie ever passed, Mae would still come up here to see Ari and Dale. They were that close.

It was another story in my office—an unhappy one. Melva was there with a report on the probate court audit.

"They found some issues and they're pretty hot about it."

"What issues? I thought we were paid up."

"We are . . . well, kind of. Remember when the thirteen came over from Warm Heart?"

"Yeah. So?"

"They came with all that money which put them over the $2,000 limit. Remember DADS went out and spent that extra money to get them down to $2,000?"

"Of course. I couldn't believe they were nice for a change. The residents loved the new stuff."

"Yeah, but that's the problem. You see, Nala Stahl just discovered that the ones they had under supervision were never paid by Warm Heart. Most of them were delinquent by fourteen months."

"What?! How did Nala Stahl allow Warm Heart to get so far behind?"

Melva shook her head. "I have no idea, and frankly I didn't ask her. Instead, she wants us to pay $3,000 for back fees since we got the money from Warm Heart and allowed it to be spent. She said we were responsible for holding that money and making sure they got paid. Something about a constructive trust and unjust enrichment."

I threw a pen down on my desk. "That's insane. *She's* insane! We had no records showing they owed any money. How could we have possibly known that?"

"Exactly. We couldn't have and I told her that. I also told her we had to move fast to spend down the money to avoid the Medicaid cap problems. But she didn't want to hear any of it. Instead, she said there would be consequences."

"What kind of consequences?"

"I don't know. She didn't say, but she sounded eight ways to pissed. Keep in mind, only three of the original Warm Heart residents are still with us."

I slapped the desk hard. "Oh no! Gracie, Dale and Ari. This is going south fast."

"Yeah, and she's going to meet with the judge and make a decision on how to handle us. We have eighteen residents under their program, so be ready for her call. She may try to reach you directly."

I took a deep breath. "Okay, I'll be ready. Print out everything I need for that call and put it on my desk as quickly as you can. After I talk with her and see what she wants, I'll call Syp. He's great with stuff like this."

"Okay," she said standing up. "It'll be on your desk by the end of the day."

I leaned back in my chair and wondered what Nala could possibly do to harm us. Could she have me or Melva arrested for contempt of court? I seriously doubted it. Fine us? How? Tell the guardians to stop sending new residents our way? I guess they could do that, but we were almost near capacity. It would take a long time for that to start hurting. Still, I wondered . . .

The next morning I arrived at work and said my usual prayer outside against the door. Melva's report was there on my desk, ready for me to refer to it should I need it. The morning flew by without a call from Nala. At 11:30 a.m. I decided to treat myself to one of my rare lunch trips away from the home. Big Dogs was on the menu. I couldn't believe how much I was liking this place. Maybe it was the steaming buns . . .

19

I was freaking out. The phone messages were worse than I'd ever imagined possible. The terror in my DON's voice was unmistakable. It was like I'd just gotten a call saying my child was being stabbed to death. Now, my foot was shaking so hard it was difficult to keep it on the gas pedal. At least I had the long drive back to try to calm myself. Yet when I managed to get calm, I couldn't keep the image of one of the Almond Joys being hauled away out of my mind for more than a few seconds. This sent me back into another round of panic. The stress was making me dizzy. I tried breathing exercises— ones I'd learned long ago during childbirth. I did them over and over to try and restart my nervous system, and perhaps even calm down. It started to work, which helped me drive more safely and get there alive.

The moment I pulled up to the home I remember thinking two distinct thoughts: the first was control. My life was one of control. I wanted to control everything, keep it organized and in its proper place. That way there was never a surprise, or at least one I wasn't prepared to deal with. Even though I believe in God and believe He's in total control, for some reason the word 'control' *controlled* my life. The second thought was how I'd assumed I was immune from the probate court's meddling. I assumed if I'd operated a right and proper nursing home, paid all the bills and followed all the rules, my residents would not be messed with. How wrong I was! This opponent was so much greater than I'd thought possible. And now I'd have to pay the price. Or actually my poor, elderly residents would have to pay the price. I hoped I wasn't too late to fix it.

I didn't have time for the employee parking lot, so I let my SUV jump the curb near the main entrance. This would save me eight more seconds. I flung the car door open, ran through the front doors and straight to the dining area. I took one look around and couldn't believe it. The place was a disaster. Several residents were sitting at their tables sucking their thumbs (a primal sign of deep stress). Nurses and CNAs stood around wiping tears from their eyes. Chairs were turned over and tables out of place. It was worse than I'd imagined.

"What happened?!"

Cayla left a small group of bawling employees and ran towards me. Between sobs she blurted out, "It's . . . terrible. We were . . . powerless to stop them."

I grabbed her shoulders and looked directly into her eyes. "Okay, calm down. I'm here. Tell me exactly what happened."

She grabbed some tissue and blew her nose. After wiping her eyes and taking several deep breaths, she spilled out this story:

Five minutes after I'd left (which is highly suspicious), five large, male CNAs dressed in scrubs entered the building, bypassed the receptionist, and walked straight to the dining room. Since the residents were just finishing up their lunch, they were all in one place. (Another coincidence?) One of them said loudly, "Gracie Peele!"

Gracie turned her wheelchair around and maneuvered over. Stopping at a table, she put one hand on the corner and said, "I'm Gracie."

"We've come to take you to another home."

Gracie thought it was a joke or a prank of some kind. She looked back at Ari and Dale, who shrugged their shoulders. Gracie turned back around and said, "Now look here you dumb bastards, you aren't going to take me anywhere. I have rights, you know."

The CNA replied, "You can say whatever you want, but we're taking you and we're doing it now." Two of the CNAs went behind and grabbed a hold of her wheelchair handles. Gracie gripped the table with both hands and held on with all her might. One of the CNAs behind her forcefully grabbed her shoulder. She lowered her head and put her mouth between his thumb and forefinger, biting down hard.

"Ooowww!" the CNA howled. He ripped his hand free of her mouth while the other hand grabbed a pile of hair, yanking her head back. That exposed her face, which was dripping blood down the corners of her mouth. The other aide jerked her hands off the table, but Gracie still didn't give up. She tried to hit his arm, but missed and instead hit the corner of the table with her thumb, splitting open her cuticle. Blood dripped out of her finger, all over the table and her dress. Gracie screamed and kicked with all her might. "No, no you bastards, you can't take me! My daughter knows where I live! I'm on the bus line where she can get to me! I can't leave! She has to know! She's all I've got!"

The two CNAs gritted their teeth and tightened their grip as Cayla and another nurse came running. "What's happening here?! You can't do that. I'm calling the police."

The lead CNA said, "Don't interfere. We have orders to take her and we're going to take her."

"I'm calling our Admin right now." (Melva just happened to be at a doctor's appointment. She wouldn't get the call until after I did.)

"I'm warning you," he barked. "Don't interfere."

Gracie tried one more time to fight them. "I have rights! I demand my fucking rights! Let me go dammit. Let me go!" One the CNAs lifted Gracie out of the wheelchair and flipped her over his shoulder. This exposed her diaper to everyone. When he turned around to take her outside, she tried to hit his arms, baring her breasts. She hadn't worn a bra in years and now all the horrified residents knew it. They carried her out upside down to a waiting van, kicking and screaming.

Back in the dining hall, some of the dazed residents rocked back and forth in confusion. A few crawled under the tables, while others ran to their rooms and slammed their doors shut. Ari and Dale were still sitting at their table in shock. Ari kept quoting over and over, "Oh, God, thy sea is so great and my boat is so small." This was way too big for him to handle. As Gracie was being hauled out, Dale quietly slipped from her chair, grabbed a hold of her walker and headed towards her room.

While Dale made her getaway, another evil CNA bent down to a resident and asked menacingly, "Where's Ari Stephenson sitting?" Fearful and shaking, the resident pointed him out. The CNA walked over and said, "Now, you're not going to give me the same type of trouble that she just did, are you?"

Ari looked straight at him and quoted Mahatma Gandhi, "Nobody can hurt me without my permission." Then surprisingly, Ari stood up and let the CNA take him to another waiting van outside.

Dale moved as fast as she could, pushing the walker hard. Sweat dotted her forehead, something that rarely happened. When she made it to the hall, the carnage of the dining room was left behind. Almost out of breath but still moving, Dale made it all the way to the entrance of her room. When she stopped and looked back down the hall, it was clear of kidnappers. Not even the residents dared show their faces. She took in a lungful of air and pushed the walker into her room. There sitting on the bed was another CNA. "I've been waiting for you," he said, smiling as Cayla came in from the hall.

"You can't take her," Cayla demanded. "I'm not going to let you!"

The man got to his feet. "Oh, I'll take her all right. And you'll be in contempt of court if you touch me or try to stop us. I have a court order. Now *stand back!*"

Tears welled up in Dale's eyes as she pleaded with the CNA. "Please don't take me. I really want to stay here."

The man grabbed her walker and turned it around pushing her from behind. "C'mon. Start walking or I'll carry you out like the other one. It's your choice."

Dale began slowly moving out, crying over and over, "Why?! Why in the Lord's name is this happening?!"

Cayla, along with Beth and Carlos, followed them out past the lobby to a third waiting van. When Dale was loaded up, the CNAs climbed in and took off. The operation was clean and quick—eight minutes from beginning to end.

When Cayla was finished with the story she stepped back and sighed. I was completely bawling, my feelings flipping between rage and sadness. I pounded the table with my fist. "Don't worry. This shall not stand! I'll get them back. You'll see."

Cayla wasn't done. "Many of the other residents are in shock. I have Dr. Lowery coming over to check them out. They think they're being taken away too. I've tried calming them down, but I have no idea if they're going to be taken away."

I blew my nose. "How's the staff?"

"Badly shaken. They felt helpless to do anything. It was like a robbery. Really, I don't know what you could've done if you'd been here."

I pounded an aching fist into my palm. "Of all the days I had to leave for lunch!" I was so filled with rage I couldn't think straight.

Another nurse came running up. "Here's something Ari left on the table as he was taken." She handed me a small cocktail napkin that said: "I will pray for you every night. And I pray that you pray for me every night."

I took the napkin and went to my office where I closed the door and had a long cry. Then I cleaned myself up and got on the phone. Billy was my first call.

"What the hell? You can't be serious!" he said. "I've never heard of something like this. Did they leave any papers?"

"No. They showed Cayla some court order, but never left us a copy. There were no discharge orders and no physician's orders.

They took no personal items, no meds, and didn't even take their records."

"Trust me Susan, no court operates like this. I've been in this business a long time. Something's wrong here. Let me get on the phone right now and call the state, see if they had anything to do with it."

"Okay, and I'm gonna call Syp."

"Good idea. You work that side and I'll work my side."

I dialed Syp's number with shaking fingers. Thankfully he picked up. "Syp, listen, three of my most precious friends in the world have been taken away from here by CNAs in three different vans. They said they had a court order, but we didn't get a copy of it."

"Shit! The red tide has reached our shores. Give me their names and let me make some calls."

I gave him the information and hung up, wiping my eyes just in time to see Melva storm into my office. "What the hell is going on?"

"Sit down and let me fill you in." When I was done she felt the same way I did. She wanted to call Nala Stahl, but I told her to hold off. I wanted to see what Billy and Syp found out first.

It wasn't until two hours later that the Aleve I'd popped started making a dent on my pounding headache. My hand still hurt, though. Dr. Lowery arrived and examined all of the residents. The anxiety level was still over the top with pills were flying out of the drug locker. He told me exactly what Billy had said, "I've been a doctor for a long time and I've never seen anything like this."

When Billy called back, he said the state had nothing to do with it. They didn't even know about it and actually doubted his story. Billy made me repeat it again so he could write down all the facts. Then he hung up to go into an emergency meeting with his executives. After all, it wasn't every day vans showed up and hauled off residents against their will.

Syp called right after I hung up from Billy. "Well kid, this is it, just what I feared. They came to harvest their organs."

"Don't say that Syp, it's not funny."

"I'm not laughing. I found out that the court *did* order them taken and they're in three separate homes. Go ahead and box up their personal affects. I'll see if I can get someone to pick it all up and taken to wherever their new homes are."

"What?! I'm not doing that. I'm getting them back and you're going to help me. That's why we have you!"

"No. My job is to solve the problems your corporate office wants solved. They're in business to make a profit and they know which battles to fight and which ones to let go. They've asked me to gather the information and nothing more. I've told you over and over, don't mess with these people. You're one court order and a doctor's opinion from being doped up yourself, drug off to a home and bankrupted. Do you want them to come back and take more residents?"

"Stop! You're helping me and that's all there is to it."

"I gotta to run." *Click.*

I called Billy back, but he was in a meeting. So I gathered up the Almond Joys' records and sat down to make some more calls. The first person I called was the guardian for Gracie.

"Listen," she said, "changing homes is the best thing for her. The Red Nine area is way too dangerous. Surely you know that."

My blood was boiling. "Why weren't you here to speak to Gracie and tell her what was going to happen?"

"Don't question me! I'm a court appointed guardian ad litem. My authority comes from a judge, not from you. Just who do you think you are?!"

"I'm somebody who gives a damn! Were you even waiting at the new home to comfort Gracie and help get her settled in?"

Click.

I called the other two guardians and the conversations were almost identical. None of them would tell me where they'd been taken or why they failed to inform their client in advance. I slammed the phone down after the last call. Melva walked in with a fax in her hand.

"The court is ordering us to erase any contact information of family or friends from the face sheet. This includes their addresses and phone numbers. We're also ordered not to contact them or their guardians."

She handed me the document. It was hard to believe this was America. "Mae!" I cried. "Poor Mae. When she comes to see her mother we won't even be able to tell her where she is. I'm going to call her up."

Melva put her hand on the phone, pushing it back down. "Don't! We're supposed to lose that information, not call them up. You'll lose your license for sure. Maybe even go to jail. Just calm down. Think this through."

"What's the harm in calling Mae? I can't just sit here and do nothing!" I was crying again.

"What is she going to do if you tell her what happened? Panic? I mean really. If you wait, Gracie may write and tell her all about this move herself." She glared at me. "Look, it's almost quitting time. Why don't you go home and get some rest. A good night's sleep will help. You'll see. Let's sit down tomorrow morning and figure out a game plan. Okay?"

I blew my nose for the hundredth time and washed down two more Aleve with a warm can of root beer. I knew she was right. My mind wasn't working properly. I turned off my office lights, grabbed my keys and left out the back.

At home, things didn't feel any better. All the adrenaline I'd been running on evaporated and left behind a feeling I'd never experienced before. It felt as if I'd swallowed a hornet's nest and every cell inside me was being viciously stung over and over again. On the outside I felt totally numb from head to toe. I needed someone to lean on, but my husband was gone. My mother and father could certainly fix this mess—they'd fixed so many in my lifetime. Yet they too had passed away years earlier. Now, I was alone, afraid, and sick inside, with no answers. The load was too heavy to carry. When the stinging sensation finally stopped, I went to the pantry and rummaged around until I found what I was looking for: a bottle of scotch. Lately I'd only been drinking with Vicki, never by myself, but this time I poured a glass and quickly downed it. I didn't even taste it. Then I downed a second. A third glass was gone like lightning. Followed by a fourth. That's when I lost count, and eventually, consciousness.

※

"Susan, wake up!" Someone slapped my face.

"W-what?"

"Are you okay?"

I tried opening my eyes and focusing, but it was difficult. Suddenly a cold, wet cloth hit my face.

"Do you think we need to get her to a hospital?" It was Vicki's voice.

"Let's give her a minute or two before we make that decision." That was Melva.

I coughed several times and opened my eyes. Vicki removed the cloth, wiping something from my mouth. "Can you understand us, Susan?"

"I couldn't save him," I mumbled.

"Couldn't save who?"

"My husband. I wasn't there for him when he was dying in my driveway."

"That was a long time ago. You're not responsible for his death."

"And I couldn't save the Almond Joys. I'm worthless. I don't deserve to be anything."

The stench of my surroundings finally hit me. Vomit was all over the couch, my clothes, the coffee table and the floor. It was terrible. I saw Vicki and Melva holding some tissue to their noses.

"Can you get up? We need to get you to the shower. Clean you up some." Vicki was urging me off the couch. I tried, but I was unsteady. Eventually, with one of them on each side, I was able to stand up and see from their point of view the carnage I'd created. It was as bad as it smelled.

I was shuffling towards the bathroom when I felt my pants sag. I'd messed myself like one of my residents. It was worse than I thought.

"What time is it?" I asked.

"It's after work," Melva said.

"H-how did you get in?" My head was spinning.

"I called Vicki when you didn't show up today. She called your son and found out where you hide the key. I met her over here and we came in together."

"So I missed a whole day's work?"

"Yeah," Melva said. "But don't worry about it. I covered for you."

I tried to break free. "I've got to dress and get in there."

"Whoa. We need to get you cleaned up and feeling better first. You're not driving anywhere. Here, drink some water."

I sipped from a glass Vicki held for me. "Now, we're going to get you undressed and into the shower. I'm bringing in one of your plastic chairs from outside and you're going to sit on that and clean up, okay?"

"Okay," I said, ready to agree to anything.

They worked with me for an hour, washing me up and getting me dressed in some comfortable clothes. I tried to throw up three more times in the shower, but nothing came up except the water I'd just taken in. Afterwards, they helped me into an easy chair in my bedroom and gave me more water to drink. Melva eventually left, leaving behind Vicki and me. With her help and the passage of time, the fog began to lift, although ever so slowly.

"Gosh, you scared us there. This is totally unlike you."

"I know. It's just that the one person who was charged to protect these three wonderful people failed. That keeps happening over and over in my life. Why?" I started to tear up.

"I don't know, but I do know you can't help get them back to your home in this condition. Melva told me all about it. She said she's working on setting up some appointments for you with the court and then you go and do this."

"Really? Okay, I'm not going to drink anymore. I'll get sober and feeling better. You'll see."

"Sure, but for tonight I want you to drink a bunch of water. When you feel like it, I want you to eat some dry toast and some yogurt. Will you do that?"

"Yes, I'm feeling better. You can leave if you want."

"I'm going to stay for another thirty minutes and make sure."

I held her hand. "You're a good friend, Vicki. Thanks for being there for me. I'm just sorry I needed you like this."

She smiled. "That's what friends do."

I shed a few more tears and drank my water until she brought me some toast along with a small plastic container of yogurt. Once I had plenty of water inside me and aspirin coursing through my veins, Vicki felt it was safe enough to leave. A few hours later I went to bed.

I still didn't feel right when I went to work the next morning, but I'd done it to myself and was blessed to not have killed myself. Alcohol poisonings kill many people each year. Plus, most of my residents had alcohol problems. I knew full well the dangers when I grabbed that bottle of scotch, yet I chose to risk my life, nonetheless. It was both stupid and reckless.

At nine o'clock, Melva and I had a meeting with Dr. Lowery. He had a long list of complaints about what had happened. "The actions of these goons injured a dozen or so residents. They're stressed out and suffering from deep anxiety. In fact, many of them are still suffering. They're afraid to leave their room for fear it's going to happen to them. This was a stupid and dangerous operation and I intend to testify to that, if need be."

"I guess you can't say anything about Gracie, Dale or Ari?" I asked.

"No, because I haven't examined them yet. I can say that separating Dale and Ari is a huge mistake. As you know, even though they aren't necessarily romantically involved, they have a co-dependency with each other. As far as Gracie goes, with the reports I heard from

Cayla and the others, I feel certain she was physically injured and most definitely psychologically harmed."

"Doctor, I'm positive you'll get your chance to testify because I'm not stopping until I get them back. Period!"

"When is the meeting?" he asked.

Melva picked up a sheet of paper and handed it to Dr. Lowery. "Next Thursday, you and Susan are meeting with Nala Stahl at the courthouse in a conference room. Here are the details."

He looked it over. "Fine. I'll have all my records together and some notes of what I want to say."

"Good," Melva said. "I think I'll get the state liaison there, too."

I slapped the table shocking everyone. "Fantastic! I'm going to have a lot to say too. Dr. Lowery, you be ready to tag team 'em."

"Don't worry, there was no medically related reason to move these three and I'm sure it caused real harm. We'll get to the bottom of this."

"All right. We just have to wait until Thursday."

It would be a long wait for me, but I was determined to have everything I needed to hit Nala the Wall hard. The guilty parties were going to pay! That was something I was sure of.

20

When Dr. Lowery and I walked into the conference room, the state liaison, Erica Gomez, was already there. So was Nala Stahl. Erica had been to our facility several times, but this was the first time she'd met Nala. It was my first time too, and my first impression wasn't heartening. She seemed a hard, bitter woman, someone with fixed opinions that rarely changed, even in the face of overwhelming evidence. A big smile suggested that she was happy to see us, yet her hand was bone cold when I shook it. We introduced ourselves and got right down to it.

Nala started. "My assistant Handy Sharpe, who handles the financial aspects of the court's program, is running a little late. We'll get started and he'll join us when he can. I understand you have some questions about the relocation of three residents."

Dr. Lowery didn't hesitate. "What was the reason for the discharge of Ari, Dale and Gracie?"

Nala smiled again. "It was the quality of the care."

"What was wrong with it?"

She frowned, acting as if she were embarrassed to have to hurt our feelings. "There were several issues. The residents weren't happy. They complained about it to their guardians. Also, the area around the home is extremely dangerous. We understand there was a knife fight recently, right out in front. It wasn't one thing really, it was a combination of things."

Dr. Lowery shook his head. "With all due respect, you're not making sense. A nurse on the scene told me Gracie fought hard *not* to leave. That doesn't sound like a person who complained to her guardian. And the area is rough, but it's been rough since the facility opened. Why now? Also, you didn't pull the other residents. I guess it's safe enough for them." He turned towards Erica. "The facility is in complete compliance with the state and has had excellent surveys recently. So now you're saying the care was not up to standard. Give me some examples." His neck was turning red. He didn't take swipes to the quality of his medical care lightly.

Nala stepped in. "Of course, I know you're upset. We hate to do this to anyone, but we felt it needed to be done. The guardians all agreed and so did the judge. They looked at everything and made this decision—a good one, I might add."

Dr. Lowery wasn't about to back down that easily. "So you have no evidence of unsatisfactory or ineffective care?"

Nala hesitated, giving me a chance to but in. "It's my facility. Did any of the guardians or the judge or you bother talking to me about any complaints?"

With a smirk she replied, "Susan, we aren't required to. If the judge had to run everything by the administrators first, the whole system would come crashing down. He trusts us to make the right decisions."

"Can we talk to the judge right now?" I demanded.

"Certainly not! He's very busy and doesn't have time for details like this. That's why he's hired me." This matched with what Syp had told me. This program was the judge's baby, but he let his staff handle almost everything. During elections, however, he trotted it out to show everyone how he was protecting the elderly and incompetent from the ravaging vultures and scam artists who preyed upon these easily-duped pigeons. His army of lawyers, guardians, banks, investors and, of course, asset managers, toiled day and night to help these tired, poor, incompetent masses, all of whom clearly yearned to be free of their financial responsibilities. And all out of the goodness of their hearts. Of course, they were able to pocket a few tiny commissions to help defray the costs of all this hard work.

Syp said Nala the Wall was the barrier between the judge and everyone else. She gave him deniability. No one could get through her to make a complaint or tell him what was going on. She was incredibly good at this and prided herself on being a 'shadow judge.' It made her feel important.

Now it was Erica's turn. "What was wrong with their care—specifically?"

"Well, like I said, it was a combination of factors." Suddenly, the conference room door opened and a man hurried in. "There you are. Everyone, this is Handy Sharp. Handy, tell them why these three residents were discharged from the Jones-Simms Nursing Center."

He plopped down in a chair and set a folder in front of him. After a heavy sigh, he looked at each of us and said, "It was financial. You folks didn't make sure we were paid, so we had to move them."

The room was so quiet, I could hear everyone breathing.

Erica cried out, "Do you understand that the residents have rights?"

Confused, Handy stood up and said, "Oh, I have their rights." He pulled a laminated square out of his shirt pocket. "See, they're right here. I keep them with me at all times."

Erica rose to her feet and pointed a finger at both Nala and Handy. "Those rights don't belong to you! You're the voice of the residents, the same residents who have those rights. Their voice is heard through you. How dare you deny anyone their rights!"

Nala stood up and moved next to Handy. "Let me tell you about your rights. You have the right to leave before I call in the bailiff. Nobody talks to us like this." With that, she forcefully grabbed a stunned Handy and left.

Erica turned to us and said, "Don't worry, I'm going to draft a report and submit this to my boss. We'll get the whole truth out and make sure this never happens again."

"Is it possible to get Ari, Dale and Gracie back while all this is going on?" I asked.

She shook her head. "I don't have that authority, but I assure you I'll talk to my boss and see what he says."

We all walked out together and for the first time since this all began, I felt like something was going to get done.

Back at the home I filled in Melva. Like me, she was very optimistic and continued working her sources for information. I went and checked on the Almond's Joys' rooms. At the time, none of them had roommates, so they had the entire space to themselves. The day everything happened I ordered their rooms not to be touched—I knew they were coming back. Besides, no one had come for anything, either.

I went into Ari's room first. I wanted to make sure my staff had followed my instructions and that everything was still in place, ready for his return. The first thing I noticed was a book of quotations on the nightstand. He had a piece of paper folded up, acting as a bookmark. I opened it up, unfolded the paper and read it. I recognized his handwriting. One line had, "You are a big part of my yesterday - Steven Tyler of Aerosmith." Another one had, "In the end, it's not the years in your life that count. It's the life in your years – Abraham Lincoln." Below that was another Lincoln quote: "Whatever you are, be a good one." I put the bookmark back in its place and returned the book to the nightstand. That's when I noticed his baseball glove. It was sticking out from under his pillow. He must have slept with it at night. There was a photo of his wife when they were both vibrant and healthy. The smiles on their faces told the whole story. I shook my head and thought, what a good man he was—*is*.

I moved on to Gracie's room. It was typical of her personality: stuff everywhere. When she was done with something, she put it down close to where it belonged and left it. Cleanliness and organization were not her strong suit. I spied the can opener hanging from a pushpin in her wall. Something was written below it: "Open yourself up to the possibilities of this world. Ari Stephenson."

Dale's room was the exact opposite of Gracie's: everything neatly put away and easy to find. Her intelligence was on display. And so was her business card, the only thing she had to show from a lifetime of work. Unlike the others, she had no photos on display. Her daughter made that impossible. The split was deep and harsh. I recalled Dale telling me that when she was at Warm Heart and the first Mother's Day came along, she received a box of chocolates in the mail from her daughter and assumed she was trying to patch things up. When she placed a piece in her mouth she had to spit it out because it was so old. When she inspected the date on the package, it was two years out of date. She told me it was a message: getting old makes things worthless. Now she was gone. I closed the door and went back to my office. All I could do was wait and see if something would be done to right this terrible wrong.

Two days later I received a call from Erica Gomez. She told me her boss wanted to meet me at the DADS office next Monday. I could hardly wait. I'd seen how outraged Erica was. I knew her boss would feel the same way.

The time passed slowly, but Monday finally arrived. I walked into the room and introduced myself to a man standing near a screen. He offered his hand. "I'm Barry Capp. Please, take a seat."

I found one and set my notes on the table. Lights clicked on illuminating the screen behind him. He had a laser pointer and turned it on, too. When he pressed a button on a clicker, a diagram appeared on the screen. At the top was a picture of a courthouse. Right below that was a photo of the Health and Human Services building where DADS had their offices—the place we were at right now. At the very bottom was a drawing of a nursing home. He aimed the red dot at the top.

"See this? This is the court." He lowered the dot to DADS. "Right below the court is us, the state." Then he moved the dot to the last image. "And this is where you are, the nursing home."

The last time I'd seen something like this was when Ross Perot ran for the presidency. I felt like a child then and now. He looked at me for a reaction and although I was burning inside, I showed none. "Now Susan, you're going to have to understand you're on the bottom tier. We're above you and the court is on top. Understand?"

I could barely speak. "So not a damn thing is going to be done about this, is it?"

"No, not a damn thing. You're just going to have to get over it," he said slamming the pointer down.

"So ripping those three great people from my home and violating all of their rights is okay?"

"If the court ordered it, their rights aren't being violated. Understand?"

I shook my head in disgust. I glanced at Erica and she looked distressed. She was staring at the table, refusing to make eye contact with me. I could tell she didn't agree with her boss, but had no power to change anything. One thing I'd learned through all my years was when to stop wasting time. This man had told me all I needed to hear. I gathered up my things and left without saying another word. When I reached my car I started crying again. I just wanted them back. They were like family to me, and losing not one, but all three of them at the same time was killing me. Now I had to face reality—they might be gone for good. Sure, I could make inquiries and try to find out which home they'd landed at. There were only sixty or so homes in the area. It wouldn't take long to find at least one of them. But what would happen if the judge found out? Would he make an example of me? Did I want to test it?

I was just about to give up when I realized I had one more card to play: Syp. In the nursing home industry, he could move mountains. I decided to drive to his home unannounced. When he opened the door, he was shocked to see me.

"Come in before they see you here!" I slipped past him as he slammed the door shut, locking it twice. "You're not going to leave it alone, are you?"

"I refuse to give up. I was entrusted with these three beautiful people and they were hurt over a measly $45. It's not right."

"No, it isn't right. But lots of things aren't right. People are starving to death all over the planet. Other people don't have clean drinking water and are dying from dysentery. Good folks are getting shot and raped right now. Are you going to fix all of them?"

"I don't have to. I only have to fix the ones in my little corner of the world. If everyone did that, what a wonderful world this would be."

"Okay, Sam Cooke. What a wonderful world it *would* be. But I have a different vision of the future. A more realistic one. Are you ready?"

"Okay."

"Remember the end of that first Indiana Jones movie, Raiders of the Lost Ark?"

He seemed to watch a lot of movies. "Sure."

"Once the probate court orders you placed in a guardianship, you're just a unit, a piece of merchandise to be measured, boxed up and stored somewhere, like in the end of that movie. And the folks who supervise the warehouse—the judge, the court personnel? They care only about how much it costs to store you. If they want to move the box to a cheaper warehouse, there's nothing you can do to prevent it. If you try, you're gonna find out how much power these folks have."

"I'm going to try anyway."

For the first time ever, he reached over and grabbed my arm. "They are God! If you pursue this, they will crush you like a box!" He shook his head in disgust. "You still don't get it, do you?"

With tears streaming down my face, I cried out, "Why isn't anyone doing anything about all of this?!"

He rubbed his jaw and thought for a moment. "The ones that know about this want to do something, but they're keeping their mouths shut before they themselves are turned into one of those boxes. "

Once again I slammed my hand on the table. "Well I'm going to do something about it, tell someone."

He smiled. "How old are you again?"

"Sixty-one. Why?"

"More than old enough for your own guardian, don't you think?"

Sometime later, a woman appeared at the facility. She didn't have an appointment nor did she give her name to the receptionist. I had to be called out to deal with her.

"We don't allow solicitors in here, ma'am. Sorry, but you'll have to leave."

"Oh, I'm not a solicitor. I have a message from a friend."

"What friend?"

She walked up to me and whispered in my ear so the receptionist couldn't hear. "Gracie."

My eyes popped out as I stepped back to look her over again. "Come on back. Taylor, hold my calls please."

I closed the door and motioned for her to sit down. "Do you know where Gracie is?"

"I do. I'm a CNA at North Creekside Care."

"North Creekside? I know where that is. Now please tell me how she is."

"Okay, but I have a long story to tell you. I witnessed a lot of it and the nurses and staff filled in the gaps when I wasn't there. Plus, I became good friends with Gracie and got a lot of the story from her firsthand. She wanted me to find you and tell it to you. Are you ready to hear it?"

I moved a tissue box closer. "Absolutely." This girl had more education than the average CNA. I could see why Gracie chose her to find me—she was able to give me more details than perhaps anyone else. This is the story she told me:

Gracie was a mess when she arrived at her new home. Her hair was bunched up with strands sticking out everywhere. Her clothes were stained with blood and wet from all the sweat. One of the abductors rolled her into her new room where she met her room-mate for the first time. At Jones-Simms, she hadn't had a roommate throughout most of her stay (except during the Katrina emergency), so this change would be very difficult for her. She thought, however, that maybe it could be used to her advantage. She might be able to persuade her roommate to help get in contact with the administrator at Jones-Simms. She knew Susan would come and get her out of there. So maybe things weren't going to be so bad after all.

The evil CNA lifted Gracie out of her wheelchair and laid her on the bed. Pulling the sheets and covers over her, he said, "An aide will come and give you a bed bath. Now you behave so everyone can do their job."

Gracie held up her two middle fingers. "Yes, sir."

He shook his head in disgust and left the room while the room-mate giggled. "What's so damn funny?" Gracie asked.

The roommate didn't answer, but she did stop giggling and jumped off her bed. She went to her dresser drawers where she pulled out a pair of little scissors. Then she started cutting out a chunk of her short hair. She wadded the hair in to a small ball, stuck it in her mouth and ate it.

"That's disgusting. Don't do that!" Gracie had seen the name on the door and said, "Are you Darla?"

She nodded.

"How long have you been here?"

Darla lifted her skirt and mooned Gracie with her underwear still on.

"Are you loony? What the hell's wrong with you?"

Darla said gleefully, "Donkey. Donkey. Donkey do and donkey don't."

Gracie quickly realized Darla was a dementia patient. She'd seen this before. "Girl, you're off this planet." Then she turned her face to the ceiling. "Oh Jesus, help me please!"

An hour later she had her bed bath. Instead of taking her to the dining room, they brought in supper on a tray. Gracie was so hungry she ate every bite. She knew she needed to regain some energy, having spent a good deal resisting her abduction. Then she fell asleep, only to wake up three hours later and witness a horrible event. Darla went into their restroom. Because the door had been removed, Gracie had a full view of Darla wrapping up medium size balls of her own feces in toilet paper. She set them down on the edge of the sink and looked at Gracie, grinning. Gracie felt ill. She'd seen what Darla had done with her hair and had no stomach for what was about to happen. Sure enough, Darla began to smear the balls all over her mouth. Her teeth were full of it. Gracie could no longer hold down her dinner. It all came up and landed on the floor. Gracie pulled the light and yelled, "I need an aide, and I need an aide now!"

An aide came and sanitized the whole room, including the restroom. The aide tried to tell Darla what she'd done wasn't acceptable and not to do it again, yet no one knew if Darla understood any of it. The odds weren't good.

Morning couldn't come soon enough. They put Gracie in her wheelchair (after she promised to be good) and led her to the dining room where she enjoyed a hearty breakfast. While eating she noticed that a CNA had a cell phone in her pocket. The CNA inadvertently left it on a table, so after finishing her breakfast, Gracie wheeled over and snatched it up. Darla was watching all of this and started yelling, "Ring! Ring! Ring!"

Gracie held a finger up to her lips, but it was too late. The aide turned around and grabbed the phone from Gracie. "You broke your promise, so you get to sit in bed and not use your wheelchair!"

Gracie hollered back, "You stupid bitch, I have rights!"

The aide said sarcastically, "Yeah, yeah, yeah, I hear you."

As they passed Darla, she stuck out both hands and grabbed Gracie's cheeks. Gracie recoiled and yelled, "Get your damn nasty hands off me!"

The aide said, "Can't you be nice?"

"I'm always nice, you bitch."

All that day and night Gracie tried to escape the place, but was caught each time. On her third day, unknown to Gracie, a nurse called the doctor who ordered Haldol (an extremely psychoactive drug that can cause hallucinations and paranoia). Two strong CNAs came into the room and held Gracie down while the nurse injected her with it. Gracie fought, yelled and screamed during the whole ordeal, but it was no use. They got it all in her. Forty-five minutes later the affects kicked in. Gracie had never had such a powerful drug and it hit her hard. She became terribly frightened of everything and everyone, curling up in a ball on her bed. The aides pulled her arms and legs apart and sat her in a chair. She wanted to cover her face and ears because the lights and sounds bothered her, but they wouldn't let her. Darla sat down beside her, picked up a fork, and poked Gracie with it. Gracie tried to get her to stop, but she couldn't. Visions of Mae popped in and out of her head. Oh how she needed to hold her child—her one and only child. In her head she pleaded with Mae to come visit. Between hallucinations she wasn't sure if she was still at North Creekside or back at Jones-Simms. She looked around for Dale and Ari, but couldn't find them. Darla danced circles around her, laughing and playing with Gracie's hair. Gracie wanted her to stop, but the drug had such a hold of her she couldn't control anything. It was a long, terrible ride she was on and she'd just have to wait for the car to stop.

After ten brutal hours, the drug finally wore off. She thought to herself, "How could anybody prescribe such a terrible drug as that?" The aides saw all this and noted in Gracie's chart that the drug had worked and that they should continue to use it to keep her calm. But Gracie knew she never wanted it again. Little did Gracie know what was in her chart.

While her head was clear she thought that perhaps she could get a letter out to Mae. She'd seen a mailbox on the corner of the building when they were bringing her in. If she could get to that and slip a letter in, off it would go. After all, they couldn't stop the mail. Darla was out of the room getting a shower, so she had the place to herself. She slid to the side of her bed and lowered herself down. Then she crawled to Darla's dresser and raised herself up on her old knees. Frantically she opened all of Darla's drawers and found a card inside a used envelope. Gracie took a pencil lying nearby and crossed through the address on the used envelope scribbling in Mae's address instead. Inside the card she wrote, "Stranger, danger." She knew Mae would understand what that meant: she needed help. Mae had been taught this as a child and would bring help. She added, "Help Me. Mom at North Creekside Care." One of Darla's stamps fit right over the last one. Perfect!

Gracie looked around for a way to get out of the room. Her wheelchair was out of the question—it was locked in a closet. She had watched them put it in there. She spotted a shower chair just outside her door. A shower chair is made of plastic tubing and has a big hole in the middle so that a person's entire butt can get washed. And it has wheels. Gracie noticed Darla had a contraption she used to pull up her socks. With it she was able to hook onto the back of the shower chair and pull it into the room.

By now her back was killing her, but she knew she had to work through it. She had to reach Mae. It took a while for her to get into the chair, but she did it. With the envelope in hand, all she had to do was make it to the mailbox outside and she was home free.

A UPS guy walked past her to deliver a package to someone. That was it! He could drop the letter in the mailbox and she wouldn't have to risk going outside. When she saw him coming back, she used her sore feet to maneuver the shower chair to the middle of the hall and block his path. She kindly asked him to place the card in the mailbox outside and he said not to worry, he'd take care of it. She thanked him and wished she had some money for a tip, but he said that wasn't necessary; he was glad to help. She thanked him again and watched as he walked down the hall and disappeared out of view. It was a huge relief. Now she could get a good night's sleep.

She wheeled herself back to her door when an aide asked her how in the world she'd managed to get onto that shower chair. She explained she'd always had a little use of her legs and needed to use them daily or she might lose the ability. She'd just wanted to exercise them. That was all, nothing more. The aide frowned and asked her if she'd been behaving herself. Gracie said she'd been good and the aide seemed to accept her explanation. The aide went to document everything Gracie had said and what she'd just seen.

The next morning Gracie woke up refreshed. She felt like her own self again. Suddenly, two nurses appeared at the door, one of them smiling. "We're baaackk!" In her hand was a syringe full of that horrible drug. The other nurse pulled out the card Gracie had tried to mail. It had been opened. "Now we've asked you nicely to behave yourself, but you didn't listen, did you?"

Gracie teared up. "Please don't give me that drug. The side effects are terrible. Please, I'll be good. I swear!"

"Oh we know you'll be good. Now relax and take your medicine like a big girl." They injected her again.

Gracie knew she had about forty-five minutes before the hell came. All she could think about was Mae. She sobbed harder than she'd ever sobbed in her life. She simply had to get back to Mae. She repeated Mae's name over and over in her head until the paranoia and hallucinations began. It was extremely painful and exhausting. Gracie felt like she was being torn apart and her world was crashing in on itself. Pieces of her brain seemed to explode. She didn't know how much longer she could take this.

Ten long hours finally came to an end and Gracie found herself sitting beside her roommate Darla. By now Gracie had nicknamed her "the Gnat." Why? Because Gracie was always trying to swat her away. She wanted the Gnat to keep away from her. She was still feeling the dying effects of the drug when they wheeled her out for dinner.

Tonight was hash. It smelled really good and brought back some fond memories for Gracie. Hash happened to be one of Mae's favorite dishes. It was made from leftover roast beef cut up into chunks and laid in gravy with chopped onions. Small squares of peeled potatoes were thrown in and everything was brought to a nice simmer. It was comfort food, for sure.

Darla was being her loony self. She kept repeating the words: knife, spoon and fork. Knife. Spoon. Fork. Knife. Spoon. Fork. It was driving Gracie crazy. If only the Gnat would just shut up. A nice CNA who had been spending time with Gracie sat down and quietly talked to her. Gracie told her everything. She said she was glad to be off of the effects of that drug, but now she felt very different. She was still trying to figure it all out. Yet she trusted this CNA with her deepest secrets because if she was going to get out of this place, she had to trust someone. Gracie wanted the CNA to contact Susan, knowing Susan would contact Mae. One thing the drug had made her realize was that she'd never explained the concept of death to Mae. Gracie knew she couldn't take much more of this drug and wanted someone to talk to Mae about it. Hopefully she'd be able to do it herself. As they talked, the CNA noticed her pupils dilate. Gracie said there was something wrong deep inside her, like a hole was expanding. It was hard for her to explain. The CNA told her not to worry and she'd be right back.

A few minutes later the CNA returned with a nurse to find Gracie's face sideways in the hash. She had no pulse. Since Gracie had a DNR on file, they did nothing more than clean up her face, haul her body back to her bed, covering it with a sheet. After all, Darla wouldn't mind.

The nurse called the guardian and he said, "It's for the best." As he was hanging up, the nurse heard him call out, "The old gray mare is finally dead!"

"So that's the whole story," the CNA said. "One she wanted you to hear." She reached over and plucked a few tissues from the box.

I leaned back and wiped my eyes. "Poor Mae. She'll miss Gracie so much. I'm so sorry I couldn't do more to save her. Those people literally killed her."

The CNA reached into her purse. "Here, she told me if something happened to take it off her and give it to you."

I reached out and held the golden twine necklace that Mae was hoping to wear one day. The tiny diamond pendant still gleamed. I slipped it over my head and let it fall around my neck. I hugged the CNA and let her go on her way. When she was gone, I pulled out a small mirror and checked it out. The necklace shined brightly in the light of my office. I could almost feel Gracie's spirit saying, "Administrator, why are you crying about this? Get off your ass and do something about this madness! You can do it, Susan, I know you can."

I rubbed the necklace and said out loud, "Yes, I believe I can."

EPILOGUE

After the visit from the CNA, I took a few days off. I was an emotional wreck. When I got back, an employee brought me the obituary section of the newspaper. There was Gracie's name, along with the dreaded phrase "Waiting for funeral arrangements due to lack of relative information." I realized that when we crossed out all the contact information per the court order, no one knew how to contact Mae. Now, Gracie was lying in some freezer waiting to be properly buried. Could this get any worse?

It had been almost five weeks when Mae finally came to visit her mother. She walked straight to Gracie's room and, of course, didn't find her there. She looked for Dale and Ari. They weren't around either. She wondered where everyone was. Thinking that maybe they were with the administrator, she rounded the corner and walked to my office. I saw the joy on her face at seeing me—finally a familiar face. We said nothing, but simply stared into each other's eyes for a few seconds. Then she got nervous and took a seat. She thought surely I'd explain where her mother was, but her expression changed when she saw my sorrowful look.

I handed her a copy of the obituary. After reading it, she fell to her knees and cried out, "No! It's not true! No!" As she wailed, I slipped the diamond necklace over her head. Tears dripped on the floor while she placed a hand up to her neck and felt it. I put a mirror down in front of her face so she could see it, but she focused on her tear-stained face instead.

As I watched her cry for her mother, I knew I couldn't tell her the details because (a) she wouldn't fully understand them, and (b) whatever she understood, it would be too devastating. When her tears finally slowed, she rose, hugged me tightly and inexplicably ran out of the home. I never saw her again. I have no idea if Gracie was ever buried. I simply had to let it go.

I had nightmares for a long time, many of which had my husband's death interwoven with the Almond Joys. It became worse when I learned from a fellow administrator that Ari had passed away within forty-eight hours of his abduction. When they looked him over, they found written on his right hand with a black sharpie, "I wanted to say goodbye to someone." I was sure I needed professional help, yet I didn't seek it. I did manage to lay off the alcohol, however.

Seven months after this incident, the Jones-Simms Nursing Center sold to some big conglomerate and I was out of a job. I soon accepted an administrator position in a rural area, and from there hoped my healing could begin. I was able to use all that I'd learned at Jones-Simms and especially from the Almond Joys to make the lives of my residents better and more fulfilling. I strove to bring out the best in them.

One day I was questioning one of my new residents about her background when she stopped and said, "You've been getting my story down. I bet you have a story to tell."

"Yeah," I said joyfully. "I've got a story to tell about three people I lost who were very dear to me and believe me, one day I'm gonna tell it!"

She smiled and said, "I bet you will, sweetie. I bet you will."

AFTERWORD

Shortly after I saw Gracie's obituary notice, I sat down with a full legal pad and made notes on everything about the event I could remember. Anything I was fuzzy about I asked Melva and those around me to clarify. Even Vicki provided a lot of details I'd missed. I vowed to myself that I'd tell everything I knew about this dirty little court program and shine a huge light on it so that one day, someone righteous and honest would come in and review each resident to see: (a) Why are they labeled incompetent? (b) What happened to their assets? (c) Who made money off with their assets? and (d) How much did they make? Then we may get the truth. I hope it comes in my lifetime.

One thing I want to make clear, there is no doubt some people need help managing their affairs. I've seen those people. They don't know who their relatives are or what day it is. They play with their feces and have no business managing their affairs. Those are easy calls. It's the folks who fade out every now and then who are the hard calls. They're sharp 85% of time, but need a break the other 15%. Are they incompetent? Maybe. Maybe not. Then there are the folks who come to the guardianship program voluntarily, much like walking up to an alligator to pet it saying, "Nice alligator." *SNAP!* They pull back and scream, "It took off my arm!" Of course, that's what alligators do. Your leg will be next. I'd think long and hard before getting into this program and I pray you never find yourself in this situation.

For those of you who find all of this hard to believe, do a little research. Late in 2015, in North Texas, I typed into google: "Probate judge who takes people's money" and the first entry was an article titled *Gavel Guardians* by Jeff Prince. The second was *Tenderize These Birds with a Gavel* in the *Fort Worth Weekly*. The third was *In Whose Best Interest* by Jeff Prince. And the fourth was *Grabbing the Purse* by Jeff Prince. Check them out and see the real faces of the folks who have been sucked up by this scheme. Read all of these stories and see if what I wrote is the truth or a lie. You decide.

Every single day I wake up and check the obituary notices for Dale. So far she's never appeared, nor have I found out where she was shipped to. I hope I'm wrong, but I'm relatively certain she died like Gracie and Ari—quickly and painfully. That's why I check the obits.

And each day I wait for a call from Syp. When it comes, it will go something like this: "Susan, they're taking me into custody right now. Please help me! PLEASE!"

I truly wish I could've created a happy ending to keep this book from being too sad and depressing, but unfortunately I can't. That's not the way it happened. Because of my belief and love for my country, the intention for this book is to inform you of the 'cracks' in its foundation. The repair can begin with you. Hopefully, God will continue to bless The United States of America.

Should you have any comments or questions, you may contact me at ABreachofTrust2016@gmail.com. I want to hear about your stories of abduction and forced poverty.

Susan Hodges, LNFA

Made in the USA
Lexington, KY
22 March 2018